Nitrates and Nitrate Tolerance in Angina Pectoris

Workshop on Nitrate Tolerance
December 16–17, 1981
Frankfurt

M. Kaltenbach · G. Kober (Eds.)

Nitrates and Nitrate Tolerance in Angina Pectoris

With 74 figures and 28 tables

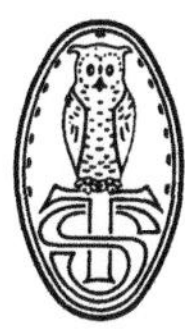

Steinkopff Verlag Darmstadt 1983

Prof. Dr. med. M. Kaltenbach
Prof. Dr. med. G. Kober
Zentrum Innere Medizin
Abteilung für Kardiologie
Theodor-Stern-Kai 7
D-6000 Frankfurt/Main 70

CIP-Kurztitelaufnahme der Deutschen Bibliothek

Nitrates and nitrate tolerance in angina pectoris / [Workshop on Nitrate Tolerance, December 16–17, 1981, Frankfurt]. M. Kaltenbach; G. Kober (eds.). – Darmstadt: Steinkopff, 1983.

ISBN-13: 978-3-642-85325-8   e-ISBN-13: 978-3-642-85323-4
DOI: 10.1007/978-3-642-85323-4

NE: Kaltenbach, Martin [Hrsg.]; Workshop on Nitrate Tolerance (1981, Frankfurt, Main).

Foreword

Although nitroglycerin is one of the oldest drugs in cardiology the problem of tolerance is a scientific challenge of today. The proceedings of this symposium highlight the most recent questions related to this topic.

Apparently, partial tolerance, or rather partial decrease in sensitivity, can arise during nitrate therapy. Probably this is the consequence of a partial readjustment of the vascular system. This readjustment refers particularly to the arterial system, i.e., to the hypotensive effect of nitrates in the standing position. A similar effect on the venous side is not present. On the other hand, the results assembled in this volume confirm the experience of many decades that long-term antianginal therapy with nitrates remains effective even when high doses are applied.

Thus partial tolerance which also occurs after other vasodilators such as prazosin, does not imply tolerance against antianginal effectiveness. From the information available today it is reasonable to treat patients with angina pectoris acutely as well as chronically with nitrates in individually adjusted doses.

Frankfurt, November 1982 M. Kaltenbach

Contents

Session III – Coronary Heart Disease

Session I:
Pharmacology

Tolerance from the Pharmacokinetic and Pharmacodynamic Viewpoints

N. Rietbrock, A. Lassmann, and B. G. Woodcock

One of the most interesting properties of many biologically active xenobiotica is that these substances not only have the capacity to stimulate a target organ but also produce desensitization or tolerance. This means that after the drug has been used for a certain time the response of the target organ disappears despite the maintained presence of the drug. This phenomenon is referred to in the literature as "desensitization", "tolerance", "tachyphylaxis", or "refractoriness". The nature of a particular receptor can be the reason why the complete spectrum of effects or a component of the drug's action is limited with respect to time on development of tolerance. If it were possible to understand the molecular basis of desensitization, then it would be possible to develop corresponding therapeutic measures. As far as can be established, only agonists have the capacity to stimulate or to desensitize a target organ; antagonists are not able to do this. For this reason it is probable that stimulation and desensitization properties of agonists are very closely correlated with one another. I should like to present the general problem of tolerance and its development and to point out the complexities of the phenomenon and its inherent molecular mechanisms – so far as these are known – using a few chosen examples. The development of tolerance can be interpreted as an adaptive protection mechanism against the effects of flooding the body with exogenous compounds or endogenous substances. Tolerance can be regarded as a very general phenomenon observable in the case of numerous substances and in conjunction with a variety of mechanisms.

One must differentiate between mechanisms causing dispositional tolerance, also referred to as "pharmacokinetic tolerance," and a genuine pharmacodynamic or functional tolerance. The cause of dispositional tolerance is a change in pharmacokinetic parameters, e.g., a reduction in absorption or an increase in the rate of elimination. An increase in the rate of elimination is, in most cases, due to enzyme induction. Changes in distribution, arising for example from a lengthening of the diffusion distance due to fibrotic changes in tissues, should also be considered. All these phenomena give rise to a reduction in the concentration at the site of action. Dispositional tolerance has little influence on the maximum response and leads in general to a decrease of no more than 30% in the original ED_{50}. Pharmacodynamic tolerance arises from adaptive changes in the receptors, so that the intensity of the response for a given concentration is reduced. Here qualitative differences in the conformation of the receptors, as well as quantitative differences concerning the number of receptors, are involved in the development of tolerance.

Alongside the classification of tolerance according to underlying mechanisms there is also a classification based upon the rate at which the tolerance develops. One can differentiate the acute form of tolerance (tachyphylaxis), which develops after a few single doses, from the chronic form, which only appears after frequent application over an extended time interval. Tolerance to opioids, alcohol, hypnotics, chlorpromazine, and weak analgesics is well known, but there are less well known examples that deserve comment.

There are several mechanisms thought to be responsible for the reduction in efficacy of the folate reductase antagonist methotrexate due to the development of tolerance. An inhibition of the transport of methotrexate to the cell, the formation of a dihydrofolate reductase enzyme analogue with reduced affinity, and an increase in the intracellular concentration of dihydrofolate reductase have been mentioned.

Irritant gases such as ozone, nitric oxides, phosgene, and sulfur dioxide in nonlethal doses produce inflammatory reactions of the alveolar-capillary barrier in the lung. These inflammatory edematous changes develop within 1–5 days and disappear within a few weeks. They increase the diffusion distance so that the inhalation of irritant gases can be repeated. The amount of gas absorbed per unit time is accordingly lower and the toxicity decreased as a result of the longer diffusion distance.

Smokers remember well how they became accustomed to the nervous and irritant symptoms that they experienced when they first began to smoke. Not only do the effects of the initial use of tobacco disappear in the case of regular smokers there is also a reduced sensitivity to the toxic effects of an intravenous nicotine infusion. This applies to the nausea, dizziness, vomiting, outbreaks of sweating and tachycardia, and also to the specific liberation of vasopressin and the characteristic changes in the EEG. Today it is well established that nicotine does not influence its own metabolism through enzyme induction, but that other components of tobacco smoke can do this and thereby accelerate the elimination of nicotine. Nicotine tolerance seems to be caused by cellular mechanisms. This conclusion is supported by experiments on mice and rats in which a clear reduction in body temperature can be observed after the first application, without any effects upon brain noradrenaline and dopamine content. After treatment with repeated nicotine injections this effect is no longer evocable, even though the nicotine content in the brain is unchanged. Up to now it has not been possible to adjust smokers for any length of time to an alternative route of application, such as oral or intravenous administration of pure nicotine. Application by way of the lungs seems to be of decicive importance for nicotine dependence following cigarette consumption. Whether or not bolus injections can lead to a flooding of the brain with nicotine and desensitization of the corresponding receptors is open to discussion, and investigation on this subject has not yet been carried out. Although nicotine causes dependence in man, in animal studies it is not as frequently self-administered as cocaine or amphetamine, indicating that nicotine is a weaker "reinforcer".

It has recently been shown in patients receiving digoxin that after a few days of treatment there are changes in the digoxin binding and intracellular sodium concentration in erythrocytes. These changes are due to the inhibitory effect of digoxin on sodium-potassium-ATPase of the cell as measured by the rubidium-86 uptake (Fig. 1). After a week of treatment only sporadic fluctuations in the digoxin binding and in the rubidium-86 transport can be observed, whereas the sodium concentration remains at the level seen after 3–4 days. In parallel the systolic time interval is shortened from 540 to 500 msec. On further digoxin application, the rubidium-86 uptake, tritiated digoxin binding, and intracellular sodium concentration return to normal values after 43 days and 140 days, respectively. Analogous observations have been made in four patient groups receiving digoxin therapy for different lengths of time (Fig. 2). The control group contained 69 patients; 38 patients took digoxin for less than 10 days; 46 patients took digoxin for longer than 2 months; and the fourth group comprised 13 patients with definitive evidence of digoxin intoxication (1).

4

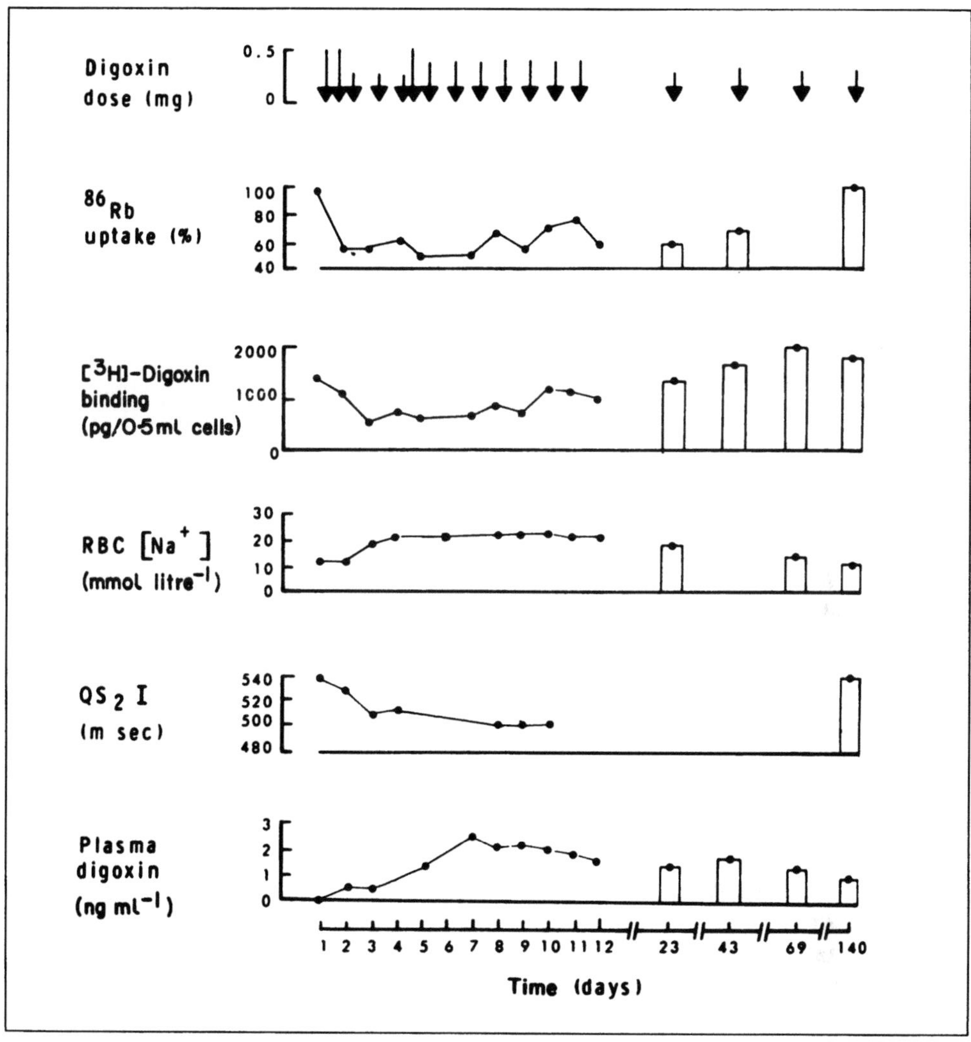

Fig. 1. Changes in rubidium-86 uptake, [3H]-digoxin binding, and intracellular Na^+-concentration of erythrocytes, QS_2I and plasma digoxin concentration in patients under short- and long-term treatment with digoxin (Aronson [1]).

The results were as follows:
1. With short-term treatment the values for the rubidium-86 uptake and the digoxin binding were lower and the erythrocyte sodium concentration higher in comparison to the nontreated group (second column, going from left to right).
2. After long-term treatment the values are no longer significantly different from those of the control group. This tolerance phenomenon is independent of the digoxin concentration level in plasma and independent of the amount of digoxin bound in vivo to the erythrocyte.
3. In some patients toxicity appeared during long-term treatment. Here the measured

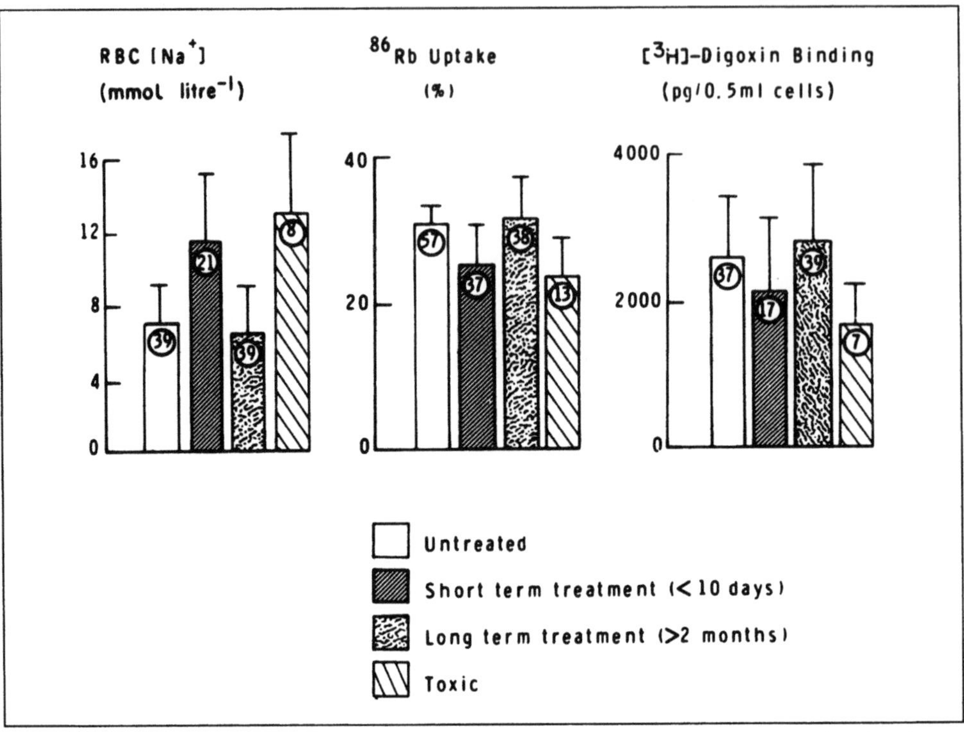

Fig. 2. Intra-erythrocyte Na⁺-concentration, rubidium-86 uptake, and [³H]-digoxin binding in red cells from four groups of patients (mean ±SD). The number of patients is indicated *on the columns* (Aronson [1]).

parameters were now significantly different from the control group and also markedly dissimilar from those in patients receiving short-term therapy.

If one could assume that the apparent pharmacological tolerance of erythrocytes during long-term therapy in some way reflected the tolerance of heart muscle to digitalis, then therapeutic success from long-term treatment of these patients would be seen as unlikely and the risk of producing digitalis intoxication could be avoided. It is known that discontinuation of digitalis treatment in some patients does not produce a worsening of the clinical condition. This applies particularly to those patients who have subtherapeutic concentrations over long periods or for whom digitalis was indicated on secondary grounds, e.g., anemia or thyrotoxicosis. These results are not unexpected. In the case of a certain percentage of patients not accurately known, and for whom there is so far no exact information available, it is possible to discontinue digitalis administration even where the serum concentration is in the therapeutic range without this procedure resulting in a worsening of the cardiac insufficiency.

From investigations on the isoproterenol stimulation of the adenylate cyclase system in frog erythrocyte membranes and the use of binding studies with [³]H-dihydroalprenolol to measure the ligand concentration, insight into the basic mechanism of beta-receptor desensitization can be gained. According to Su and co-workers (7) desensitization processes can be divided into a homologous type and a heterologous type. In the case of homolo-

6

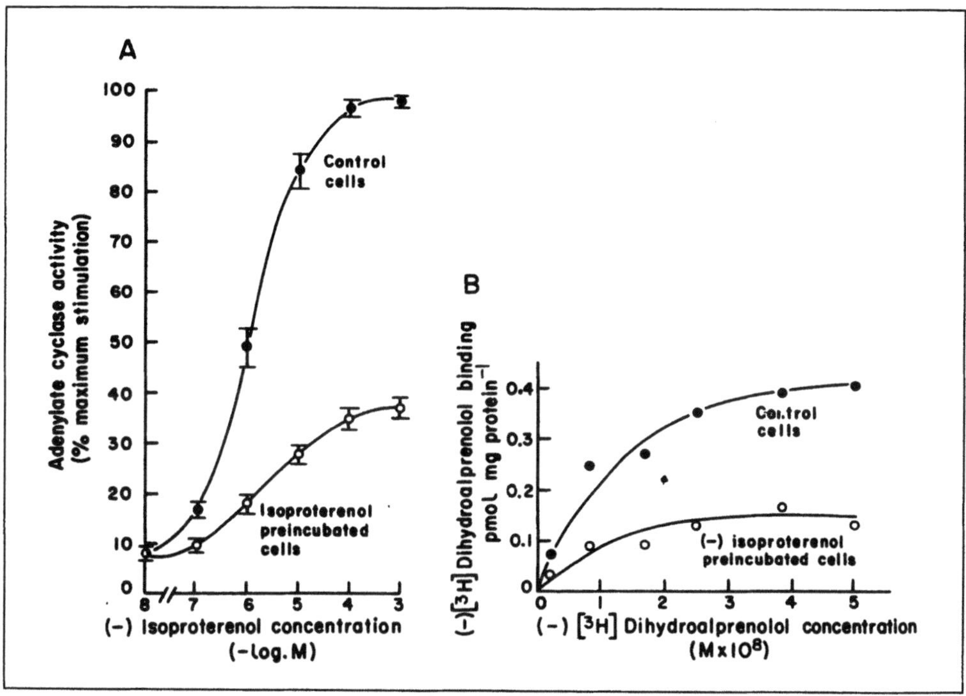

Fig. 3.a Stimulation of adenylate cyclase by isoproterenol (isoprenaline) in frog erythrocyte membranes with and without preincubation with isoproterenol. Maximal stimulation in control = 100%; equivalent to the formation of 396 ± 82 pmol cAMP/mg · min⁻¹ (Mickey et al. [5]); **b** specific binding of (–) [³H]-dihydroalprenolol as a function of the ligand concentration in frog erythrocyte membranes with and without preincubation with isoproterenol.

gous desensitization, the incubation of receptor cells with an agonist leads to a reduction in excitation in response to the agonist itself and in response to structurally similar substances. In the case of heterologous desensitization, exposure to an agonist leads to a reduction in excitation not only with the agonist but also with other types of stimulatory substance having widely different structures. Figure 3a) shows the fundamental aspects of the catecholamine-induced homologous desensitization of frog erythrocytes. If cells are exposed for a period of minutes, or in some cases hours, to a beta-adrenergic catecholamine, there occurs a progressive reduction in the stimulatory effect of isoproterenol on adenylate cyclase activity associated with the beta-receptor. It can be seen from Fig. 3b) that, using the specific beta-adrenergic blocker dihydroalprenolol, the number of available binding sites in desensitized cells decreases by 60%. Antagonists are not able to desensitize the system and do not lead to a reduction in receptor density (3).
The molecular mechanisms in desensitization are incompletely understood. The process in frog erythrocytes is slowly reversible and appears to proceed without de novo protein synthesis. Computer calculations of binding curves show that in the case of alprenolol and other antagonists a single homogeneous binding site exists (Fig. 4a), while for agonists such as isoproterenol the binding site has two interconvertible states, one with high affinity (H) and one with low affinity (L). Twenty-five percent are of the low-affinity type

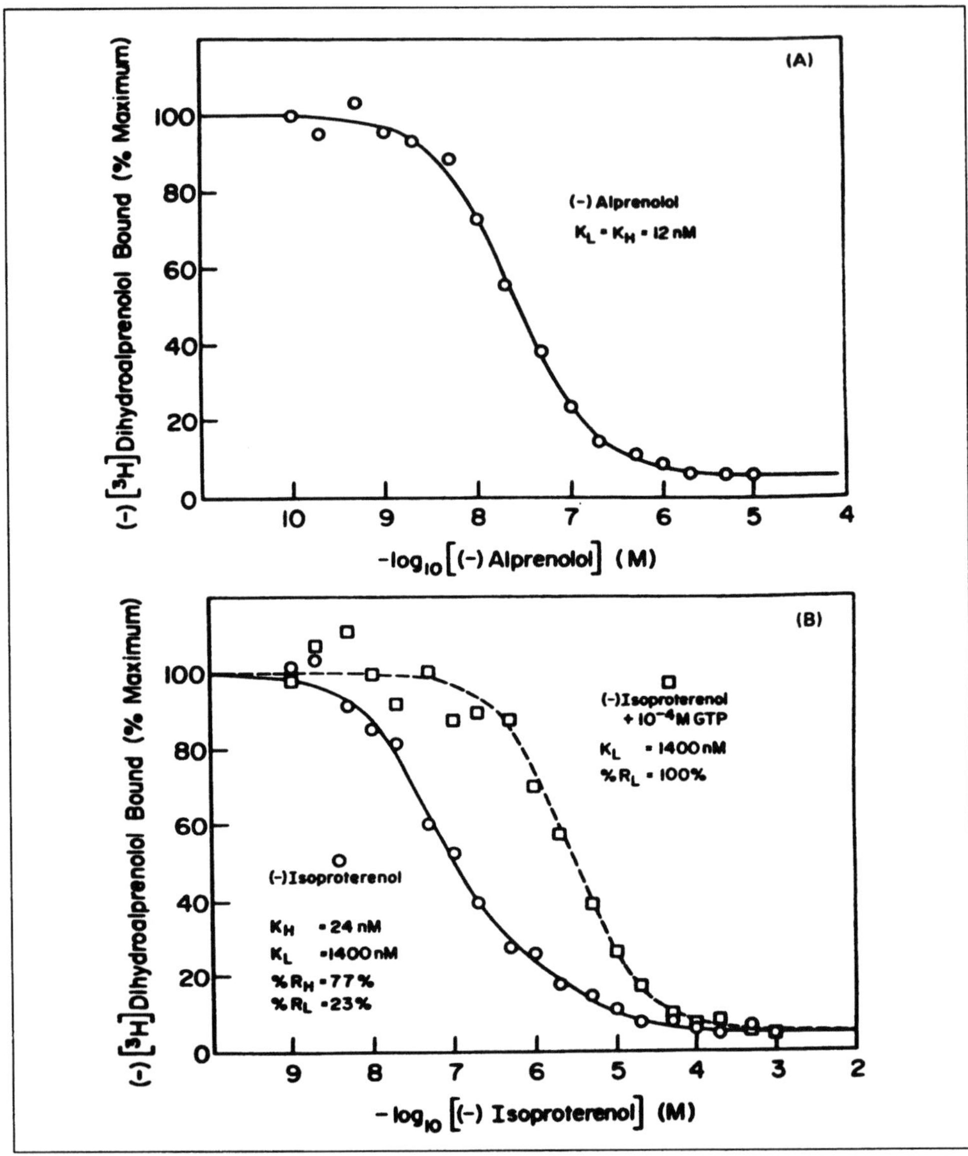

Fig. 4.a Fitted curve showing the displacement by (–) alprenolol as a percentage of maximal binding of (–) [³H]-dihydroalprenolol bound to frog erythrocyte membranes. *H*, high-affinity type site; *L*, low-affinity type site (Kent et al. [2]); **b** Fitted curve showing the displacement by isoproterenol of bound (–) [³H]-dihydroalprenolol in frog erythrocyte membranes with and without guanyl nucleotide (*GTP*). *H*, high-affinity type site; L, low-affinity type site (Kent et al. [2]).

and 75% of the high-affinity type (Fig. 4b). The ratio of the corresponding dissociation constants K_L and K_H is approximately 60 : 1. In the presence of a high concentration of guanine nucleotide (10^{-4} *M* GTP) the binding curve is moved toward the right and is steeper. Although the total number of binding sites remains the same they are all now the

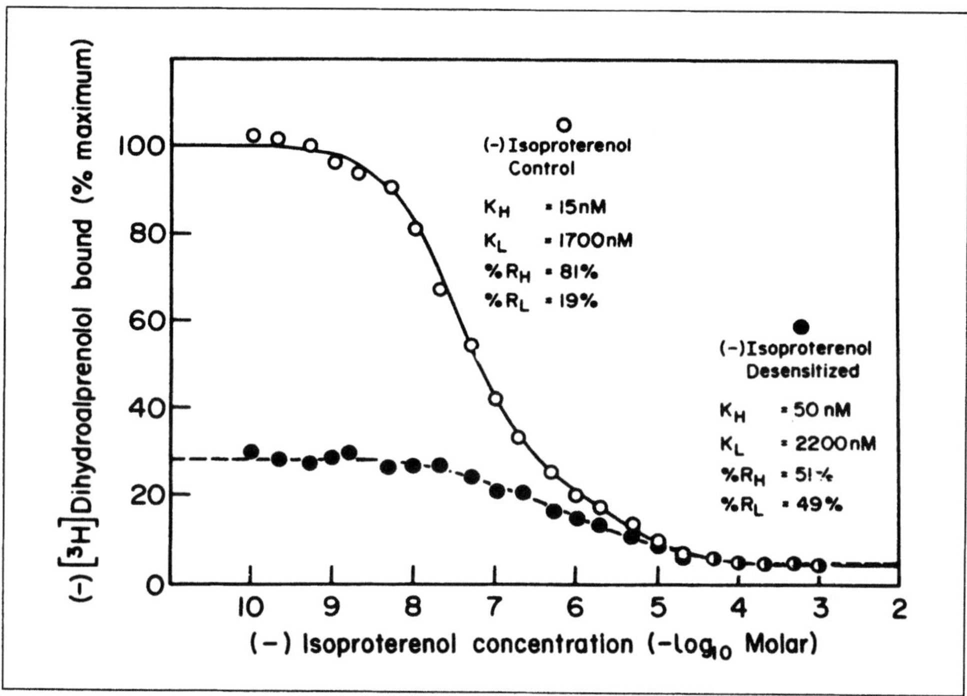

Fig. 5. The expression of desensitization on the concentration of high-(*H*) and low-(*L*) affinity type receptor-binding sites. The total decrease in the maximum (–) [³H]-dihydroalprenolol binding was 70%. The decrease (± SEM) in the binding sites with high affinity from 81% to 51% was significant (Kent et al.[2]).

low-affinity type (4). The results of a further study (Fig. 5) show several alterations in the receptors of desensitized frog erythrocytes (2). The number of dihydroalprenolol receptors is decreased by approximately 70% in comparison with normal cells, so that less dihydroalprenolol is bound. The dissociation constant K_H for isoproterenol increases from 15 n*M* to 50 n*M*, and K_L from 1700 n*M* to 2200 n*M*. The ratio $K_L:K_H$ is reduced from 113 to 44.

The agonist is only able to stimulate the receptors in the high affinity state. Desensitization leads not only to changes in the interaction between agonist and receptor but also to an actual reduction of receptors.

Clearly, receptor-binding studies are vital and effective tools that can help to unravel the complex processes comprising tolerance. There exist numerous clinical data on nitrate tolerance. In the main they are derived without regular measurements of nitrate concentration in blood with respect to time. It is not surprising, therefore, that they cannot exclude the involvement of a pharmacokinetic basis. Owing to insufficient basic knowledge about the processes at receptor level, there is much controversial discussion on the nature of nitrate tolerance.

Reports on nitrate tolerance include objective parameters such as heart rate, blood pressure, blood flow, vascular resistance, heart minute-volume, mean pulmonary artery pressure, and ST-segment depression, among others, as well as subjective information from the patient, such as frequency and severity of anginal attacks and nitrate headache.

It should be noted that in most cases nitrates remain active over months and years, and a falling-off in efficacy can only be observed in the occasional patient.

Those who deny the reality of nitrate tolerance make references to the type of illness and cause of disease. Coronary stenosis due to arteriosclerotic changes or raised vascular tone or thromboembolic processes, an advancement of the underlying illness, noncompliance, omission of concentration measurements, counter-regulatory or homeostatic mechanisms, and insufficient experience in the use of the drug have been mentioned. The proponents claim that nitrate tolerance exists independently of the type of nitrate used and the nature of the galenic formulation. The arguments are based on investigations that are worthy of attention but at the same time fragmentary. The methodology and the statistical analysis of many studies leave much to be desired. If one postulates that organic nitrates behave as agonists at the receptor level it can be understood why blood vessels from animals made tolerant are found to be desensitized in vitro and are much less responsive to nitrates. Furthermore, Needleman and Johnson (6) have suggested that oxidation of critical sulf-hydryl groups on nitrate receptors of vessels occurs, and that these can regain their sensitivity on treatment with dithiotreitol. These results should encourage the carrying out of further intensive investigations in order to reconcile clinical experience with fundamental pharmacological knowledge.

Tolerance is not a universal phenomenon. It is always selective since not all responses are uniformly affected. Tolerance is often defined as a decrease in response to a given dose, even though it is pointed out repeatedly that the use of this definition makes it impossible to differentiate between a movement to the right of the dose-response curve and a reduction in the maximum effect without change in the ED_{50}. A movement to the right in the dose-response curve can as readily be attributed to pharmacokinetic as to pharmacodynamic causes. That is to say, a lower blood concentration is obtained for a given dose or there is a change in the response of the receptors. A differentiation in these cases is only possible when the clinical efficacy is viewed in relation to the measured concentration.

The tolerance phenomenon is observable at all biological levels: for example, in the enzyme constitution in single cells and subcellular units, and in the metabolic control and physiological function of an organ or the whole body. Tolerance phenomena are normally encountered with respect to easily diagnosed subjective complaints or specific clinical responses. The interpretation of these observations depends on the standpoint of the investigator. Pharmacologists, clinicians, and chemists will try to approach and explain tolerance phenomena differently.

One may be sure, that with time, proponents and opponents of the tolerance theory will agree with one another since they both seek the truth. In everyday conversation "tolerance" can frequently be substituted for "patience". For the moment one must ask for tolerance in regard to tolerance.

References

1. Aronson JK: The effects of digoxin on red cell digitalis receptor function in man. In: Clinical Pharmacology and Therapeutics, p. 135. Proceedings of the first world conference 1980. Ed P Turner, MacMillan Publisher Ltd, London and Basingstoke.
2. Kent RS, de Lean A, Lefkowitz RJ: A quantitative analysis of beta-adrenergic receptor interactions: Resolution of high and low affinity states of the receptor by computer modeling of ligand binding data. Mol Pharmacol 17: 14 (1980).

3. Lefkowitz RJ: Mechanisms for regulation of β-adrenergic receptor function in desensitization. In: Clinical Pharmacology and Therapeutics, p. 145. Proceedings of the first world conference 1980. Ed P Turner, MacMillan Publisher Ltd, London and Basingstoke.
4. Lefkowitz RJ, Hoffman BB: New directions in adrenergic receptor research. Part I. TIPS, Vol 1, p. 314 (1980).
5. Mickey JV, Tate R, Lefkowitz RJ: Subsensitivity of adenylate cyclase and decreased β-adrenergic receptor binding after chronic exposure to (−) isoproterenol in vitro. J biol Chem 250: 5727 (1975).
6. Needleman P, Johnson EM jr: The pharmacological and biochemical interaction of organic nitrates with sulfhydryls. In: Organic nitrates. Needleman P: Ed Handbuch der experimentellen Pharmakologie, Vol 40, Springer-Verlag, Berlin 1975, pp. 97–114.
7. Su YE, Cubeddu L, Perkins IP: Regulation of adenosine 3': 5'-monophosphate content of human astrocytoma cells: desensitization to catecholamines and prostaglandins. J cyclic Nucl Res 2: 257 (1976).

Authors' address:
Dr. N. Rietbrock
Zentrum der Pharmakologie
Abteilung für Klinische Pharmakologie
Theodor-Stern-Kai 7
6000 Frankfurt 70

Does Tolerance Develop During Long-Acting Nitrate Therapy?
A Critical Review

Jonathan Abrams

Introduction

Nitroglycerin and long-acting nitrate esters are playing an increasingly wide role in medicine. These agents are effective in the treatment of a variety of cardiovascular conditions (Table 1) and are the mainstay of therapy in the medical treatment of angina pectoris. Many patients with moderately severe congestive heart failure benefit from nitrates, with reductions in left-ventricular filling pressures and maintained or increased cardiac output. During the past 5–7 years it has been shown convincingly that high-dose nitrate therapy is often necessary, particularly in heart failure or refractory angina. Many patients are now receiving nitrates in amounts that formerly would have been considered excessive, but are actually necessary to provide adequate bioavailability and sustained pharmacological activity (1, 2).

Pharmaceutical companies around the world have developed a wide array of nitrate delivery systems (Table 2) designed to make it easier for patients to use these drugs and to provide sustained therapeutic levels of nitrate esters in the plasma.

In light of the increasingly widespread application of high-dose nitrate therapy, the question of nitrate tolerance becomes a critical issue. Tolerance is well defined by Rietbrock et al. elsewhere in this symposium; in essence, it means that a drug becomes less effective or even ineffective over time. Typically, increasing amounts are required to maintain a given therapeutic effect. Of potential importance to nitrate therapy, tolerance is more likely to develop with larger doses of a drug. Tolerance is often incomplete, and there may be different degrees of tolerance to the various actions of a given agent. Cross-tolerance to related compounds may appear, and is particularly relevant to the use of

Table 1. Usefulness of nitrate therapy in Cardiovascular disease.

Typical effort-induced angina pectoris

Coronary vasospasm
  Unstable angina syndromes
  Prinzmetal's variant angina

Acute and chronic congestive heart failure in patients with elevated left-ventricular preload and low cardiac output.

Acute myocardial infarction
  Decreased chest pain and ST-segment elevation
  Reduction of infarct size
  Decrease in malignant ventricular arrhythmias

Control of blood pressure during general anesthesia.

Evaluation of left-ventricular wall motion disorders during left-ventricular angiography.

Table 2. Nitrate delivery systems (*NTG,* nitroglycerin; *ISDN,* isosorbide dinitrate).

Sublingual	NTG	ISDN
Chewable		ISDN
Oral	NTG	ISDN
Buccal	NTG	
Nasal spray	NTG	
Oral spray		ISDN
Topical (ointment)	NTG	ISDN
NTG-impregnated disc	NTG	
Intravenous	NTG	ISDN

nitrates, where many patients on chronic long-acting therapy also use sublingual nitro-glycerin or isosorbide dinitrate (ISDN).

Evidence for Nitrate Tolerance

Tolerance to nitroglycerin and long-acting nitrates has been well documented. The earliest reports date back to 1888 (3). I recently reviewed much of this evidence (4, 5), which comes from animal studies (4, 6, 7) as well as investigations in human subjects (4, 8, 9). Most of these studies conclude that nitrate-induced reduction in arterial resistance and systolic blood pressure may rapidly disappear with chronic dosing. One recent study, however, found that the venodilatory effects of nitroglycerin became attenuated after 6–8 weeks of oral ISDN but that the arterial actions remained intact (10). In vitro studies indicate that vascular smooth muscle can become completely unresponsive to nitroglycerin after exposure to organic nitrates (11).

While it is true that counterregulatory mechanisms (e.g., increased sympathetic activity, resetting of baroreceptors, etc.) may account for much of the attenuation of nitrate effects on blood vessels during chronic treatment, the experimental work of Needleman suggests that nitrate tolerance can be initiated with a single dose (11). His study using isolated aortic strips indicates that compensatory vasoconstriction in intact subjects cannot completely account for the disappearance of hypotensive activity after chronic nitrate treatment. Nevertheless, when I initially reviewed this subject, I concluded that the overwhelming evidence indicated that nitrate tolerance is not a problem in clinical medicine (4). Many well-conducted contemporary trials in angina pectoris and congestive heart failure have clearly demonstrated continued responsiveness to the beneficial actions of nitrates after chronic dosing.

The fact that this workshop on nitrate tolerance has been convened indicates that my initial assessment may need modification. This has come about mostly because of the recent work of Thadani and Parker (12–14), who carried out an investigation in angina patients who were given ISDN in varying doses over a period of weeks and were found to develop tolerance. Investigators in West Germany have also suggested that nitrate tolerance is a real problem (15). The old dilemma is again at hand and requires a careful reevaluation at this time.

The rest of this chapter will be devoted mainly to work that has been carried out since 1979, in an effort to update my previous reviews (4, 5).

Recent Evidence Favoring Tolerance

Thadani and Parker's study is without doubt the most important investigation supporting the development of nitrate tolerance. In a group of 12 patients with chronic stable effort angina they demonstrated that short-term oral treatment with ISDN, even 15 mg four times a day for 1 week, rapidly induced an attenuation of nitrate actions (12–14). In a double-blind protocol all patients were initially studied acutely with individual ISDN doses of 15, 30, 60, and 120 mg, as well as placebo, with at least 1 day between each study. The subjects were then given placebo for 2 weeks and subsequently treated with increasing amounts of ISDN in the same dosages, with each level of nitrate administered four times a day for 1 week (single-blind protocol). Heart rate and blood pressure were measured continuously for 8 h in the supine and upright positions, and serial treadmill exercises were performed at 0, 2, 4, 6, and 8 h at each ISDN dose in both the acute and chronic phases of the study. Isosorbide dinitrate blood levels were measured as well. The results summarized below clearly indicate the development of partial hemodynamic tolerance to ISDN, with a marked reduction of the magnitude of heart rate responses to nitrate and decreased duration of action on blood pressure from 8 to 4 h (Fig. 1):

1. Acute effects of ISDN on blood pressure and exercise tolerance were dose-related and lasted 6–8 h.
2. Circulatory tolerance to repeated dosing rapidly appeared (within 24 h) with attenuated systolic blood pressure responses, decreased duration of effect to 4 h, and abolition of any increase in heart rate.
3. Improvement in treadmill exercise duration decreased from 6 to 2 h after repeated ISDN administration.
4. Cross-tolerance to sublingual nitroglycerin occurred with respect to blood pressure and heart rate responses.
5. During chronic therapy with ISDN the dose–response relationship with respect to blood pressure, heart rate, and exercise duration was no longer apparent, and higher doses of ISDN had little additional therapeutic effect.
6. Plasma ISDN levels were higher after chronic dosing.

Of greater importance was the shortened duration of nitrate-induced exercise improvement, as well as the disappearance of any obvious dose–response effect (14). Angina protection, as evidenced by treadmill-walking time to onset of angina as well as to angina of "moderate severity," was fully 8 h for all four dose strengths in the acute phase, but lasted only 2 h after "chronic" treatment with ISDN at any dosage level. In addition, the improvement in ischemic ST-segment response noted in the acute stage was no longer apparent (14). These results could not be attributed to an increase in ISDN metabolism or other pharmacokinetic alterations, in that ISDN blood levels were actually higher after chronic dosing (13). This is consistent with Needleman's previous work, which excluded biotransformation or enhanced excretion of nitrate as possible mechanisms for tolerance (6, 7).

These data are somewhat discordant from the earlier studies of Lee et al. (15) and Danahy et al. (16). Danahy found no decrease in treadmill time up to 3 h following ISDN in angina patients treated for 3–10 months; however, ISDN was not found to be effective at 5 h. Attenuated heart rate and blood pressure responses after chronic dosing with ISDN were noted.

Cross-tolerance to nitroglycerin was not evaluated in Danahy's earlier study, as it was in the study of Thadani and Parker (13). The latter examined heart rate and blood pressure changes following sublingual administration of nitroglycerin and did not investigate

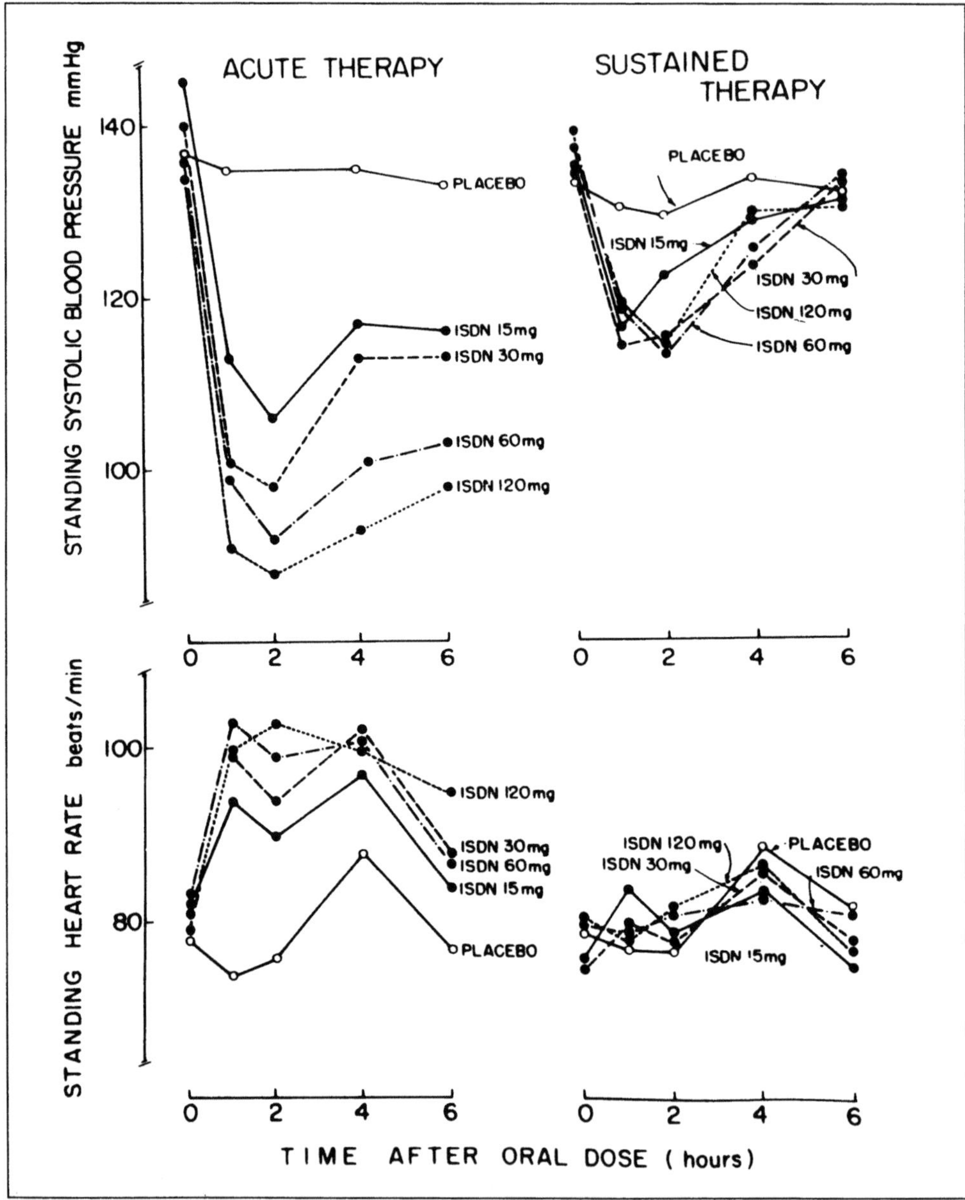

Fig. 1. Standing blood pressure and heart rate data in acute and sustained therapy (mean values taken from six patients). Note that the changes in blood pressure and heart rate seen with acute dosing are attenuated after sustained therapy. Systolic blood pressure still decreases significantly after each dose compared to placebo, but the effects in reduction of blood pressure lasted only 4 h. There were no significant increases in heart rate following isosorbide dinitrate (ISDN) during chronic therapy. Thadani et al. 1980 (by permission of the American Heart Association).

16

whether the enhanced exercise capacity produced by nitroglycerin was altered by chronic ISDN therapy. In Lee's study no loss of maximal sublingual nitroglycerin efficacy was noted after 1 month of ISDN (40 mg four times a day) therapy; cross-tolerance was not documented. Although the exercise increase following sublingual nitroglycerin was somewhat less than before ISDN treatment, the maximal treadmill performance following ISDN was similar before and after 1 month of ISDN therapy. However, this protocol did not specifically examine whether tolerance to ISDN itself developed, as the subjects were rechallenged only with sublingual nitroglycerin, and at least 6 h or more following the last dose of ISDN. Baseline exercise duration was greater in the ISDN group after 1 month, clearly suggesting a duration of effectiveness of ISDN greater than 6 h, but this protocol did not involve repeat dosing with ISDN and subsequent assessment of exercise response after ISDN. Thus this investigation does not actually contradict the work of Thadani.

It is not clear that the differences in duration of the protective effects of ISDN (3 h (16) versus 2 h (14)) are very important, given the major difference in protocol design between the three studies. Only the Ontario group carried out stress tests for as long as 6 and 8 h after ISDN; while their acute study showed a protective effect of ISDN with respect to treadmill time at 4, 6, and 8 h after dosing, most previously reported investigations with ISDN have shown a briefer duration of action of 2–4 h (18).

Rudolph et al. have reported a study in patients with angina given slow-release ISDN for individual periods of 8 weeks who showed no clinical benefit at a dosage of 20, 40, or 60 mg three times a day when tested 3 h after dosing (18). In this protocol each individual subject was apparently not tested acutely with ISDN and then subsequently shown to loose the protective response with chronic dosing. A related investigation did show blood pressure, heart rate, and ST-segment responses to the acute administration of ISDN that lasted 8 h (18). Although nitroglycerin consumption, heart rate, and blood pressure responses were not altered by oral treatment with ISDN, the protocol does not specifically document the development of tolerance in the test subjects. Rather it indicates a lack of effectiveness of orally administered ISDN in this group of patients. Many other well-designed studies with ISDN have clearly documented sustained antianginal protection with long-acting nitrates (17, 19) and this negative study should be placed in this broader perspective.

In this symposium Tauchert and Hombach report a study that supports the development of tolerance to nitrates (20). Using oral administration of isosorbide-5-mononitrate they demonstrated a failure of the nitrate to protect against exercise-induced elevation in pulmonary artery pressure after 3 weeks of therapy with 50 mg three times a day in patients in whom the drug did prevent exercise-induced pulmonary artery pressure increases following acute administration. Exercise duration, ST-segment response, and time to angina were not reported. It is therefore unclear what the implications of this study are with respect to clinical tolerance. They suggest that the sustained concentrations of the 5-mononitrate may have contributed to the development of tolerance. Others have postulated that brief interruptions of nitrate therapy may protect against tolerance, and previous animal studies have demonstrated that tolerance readily disappears after cessation of nitrate administration, with a subsequent complete recovery of vascular responsiveness. The temporal relationships of nitrate plasma and tissue concentrations to nitrate tolerance need to be vigorously pursued in future investigations.

Recent Studies Not Supportive of Nitrate Tolerance

In addition to a number of previously reported trials that did not find evidence for nitrate tolerance, including the only systematic evaluation of nitrate tolerance in congestive heart failure (21), several recent studies have been completed that do not confirm the phenomenon of tolerance. Becker et al. first reported the absence of nitrate tolerance in angina patients given 100 mg ISDN daily for up to 9 weeks, with repeat treadmill evaluations and assessment of ST-segment depression at a fixed workload using acute doses of 10 mg or 30 mg ISDN (22). Recently he has reported the absence of tolerance in one group of patients given 60–160 mg ISDN per day for 6 months (23) and in another group of patients who have been taking ISDN for up to 5 years (24). The subjects were given treadmill tests after both ISDN and placebo. No tolerance was found in either group. One methodological criticism is the cessation of ISDN treatment for at least 24 h before rechallenge; this nitrate-free interval conceivably could have restored vascular responsiveness. Schneider et al. found that high-dose ISDN (120–480 mg/day) given six times daily resulted in sustained exercise improvement and angina protection in patients given a fixed exercise workload (25). However, there was some reduction in the ST-segment improvement after 4 weeks of high-dose ISDN therapy (480 mg daily). Compared to acute therapy, heart rate and blood pressure responses to ISDN were absent after the sustained high-dose treatment, again demonstrating the phenomenon of vascular tolerance.

In two dissimilar investigations utilizing ISDN ointment, tolerance was found to be lacking. Distante et al. demonstrated sustained responsiveness to intravenous ISDN infusions with respect to heart rate and blood pressure alterations (26). Subjects with angina were treated with 100–200 mg ISDN ointment three times a day for 12–18 months and were repeatedly tested with intravenous ISDN infusions. This group did not find the blunted circulatory changes that have been documented by numerous other investigations following chronic long-acting nitrate treatment. This was not a protocol that examined the clinical efficacy of ISDN. Brunner et al. documented antianginal efficacy of topical ISDN in a small group of effort angina patients treated with ISDN ointment (150–200 mg/day) for 6–8 months (27). These patients were exercised three times after treatment was begun at an average interval of 2–3 months between tests. Sustained improvement in bicycle ergometer time, ST-segment depression, and relief of chest pain was noted in six of eight subjects. In addition, the patients noted a decrease in nitroglycerin consumption and angina attacks over the duration of the study. All patients were also given additional sublingual ISDN at peak exercise and demonstrated further enhancement of exercise capacity, indicating a lack of cross-tolerance between the two formulations of ISDN. This study, however, did not use a fixed or reproducible test protocol among the patients, and the absence of tolerance can only be assumed from the data given. Placebo was not given at any time and only one initial baseline stress test was used for future treadmill comparisons.

In another study reported in this symposium, Distante et al. failed to find tolerance in 40 patients given ISDN orally for an average of 21 months (range 1–50) (28). Blood pressure and heart rate responses to sublingual ISDN were assessed in five groups of patients, according to duration of prior ISDN therapy. These workers could not find any significant attenuation of the increase in heart rate or decrease in systolic blood pressure with the challenge dose. These data do not address the question of group responses as carefully as other studies, but are consistent with the authors' previous findings in subjects given ISDN ointment (26). It should be stressed that this investigation did not assess angina frequency or utilize serial treadmill tests.

Niederer et al. have conducted an elegant invasive study in ten angina patients given ISDN orally for 4 weeks (29). The subjects underwent left and right heart catheterization with exercise before and after the nitrate therapy. Exercise-induced increases in left-ventricular enddiastolic pressure and pulmonary artery pressure, as well as decreases in left-ventricular ejection fraction, were blocked by acute oral administration of 50 mg ISDN. After 1 month of therapy with 180 mg ISDN daily, the subjects underwent repeat catheterization; the improved hemodynamics with exercise after ISDN were maintained, indicating the lack of development of tolerance. However, no decrease in left-ventricular systolic pressure produced by ISDN in the first study was noted at rest or exercise in the second study, suggesting tolerance development to the arterial effects of nitrate. Hauf et al. have demonstrated a continued response to ISDN in patients with congestive heart failure given a repeat challenge after 12 days of 20 mg ISDN given orally three times a day (30). These patients had no nitrate for at least 15 h before being given a much larger dose of ISDN (100 mg) than used on a daily basis. Not only did left-ventricular filling pressure fall after ISDN, but the baseline left-ventricular filling pressure had decreased significantly after 12 days of therapy.

Bassan and Weiler-Ravell carried out a careful investigation in ten patients with angina who were taking propranolol and were then given ISDN to assess the antianginal efficacy of the nitrate added to a beta-blocker (31). These patients were tested with hourly treadmill exercise for 8 h on 2 separate days after receiving placebo or ISDN in a double-blind protocol. Two of these subjects had been taking oral ISDN regularly for 1 or more years in a dosage of 100–125 mg/day. Both responded positively to oral administration of ISDN, with substantial improvement in bicycle exercise time for 4–6 h after repeat dosing; one patient still had a response at $7^{1}/_{2}$ h after receiving ISDN. The two patients also had a 20-mmHg or greater fall in systolic blood pressure when given ISDN. These data in only two patients demonstrate sustained responsiveness to ISDN after prolonged therapy for 1–3 years. This does not allow a comparison to Thadani's study in that the two patients did not have an acute dosing trial with ISDN. Nevertheless, this clearly suggests that nitrate tolerance does not necessarily develop after ISDN treatment.

Pharmacological Aspects of Nitrate Tolerance

It is clear that the question of tolerance is more complex than was previously thought. Little is known about nitrate receptor availability after acute or chronic dosing. Needleman's concept that oxidized sulfhydryl groups in vascular smooth muscle play a role in tolerance is a hypothesis that does not really elucidate all the unresolved questions (6, 7). Work from Ontario suggests that altered metabolism of nitrate does not provide a simple answer. In Thadani's study ISDN plasma levels were higher after chronic therapy than after acute dosing with the same amount of oral nitrate. Armstrong has demonstrated a decrease in the arterial–venous nitroglycerin gradient and an elevation in venous nitroglcerin levels after high-dose nitroglycerin ointment administration in dogs subsequently given an intravenous nitroglycerin infusion (32).

These animals developed attenuation in the hemodynamic response to nitroglycerin (33). This work also demonstrates that pharmacokinetic alterations in nitrate metabolism (e.g., increased metabolism, biotransformation) are not the cause of tolerance. Tissue nitrate receptor saturation, with binding of nitrate receptors or alterations in the affinity of receptors for nitrates, may play an important role in the development of nitrate tolerance.

Fung suggests that examination of nitrate kinetics within blood vessels may be far more profitable than the study of plasma concentrations and kinetics (34). He has shown that veins appear to take up nitroglycerin more readily than arterial walls on a nanogram per gram of wet tissue basis (35). This is consistent with clinical observations that nitrate effects on capacitance vessels occur at lower plasma concentrations than those required to dilate the arterial or resistance vessels. Whether this relates to the question of tolerance is speculative. Much work suggests that tolerance is more readily induced to the arterial effects of nitrate. The age-old observation of disappearance of nitrate headache attests to this. However, Zelis and Mason's study on nitrate tolerance indicated that venous dilatation is attenuated following chronic ISDN treatment but that arterial dilatation is not (10). Distante's work also suggests that arterial responsiveness is not attenuated with chronic nitrate treatment (26, 28). The literature is most confusing in this regard.

It should be pointed out that there are differing views on how nitroglycerin exerts its clinical actions. Peripheral arterial and venous dilatation with decreased left-ventricular preload and afterload have been felt to be of primary importance in reducing myocardial oxygen demands in relief of anginal chest pain. However, there is considerable work documenting the direct beneficial effects of nitroglycerin on the coronary circulation; some studies clearly support a decrease in subendocardial ischemia and improvement in regional myocardial perfusion during acute myocardial ischemia (36). The precise role of preload reduction versus systemic or coronary arterial dilatation is far from clear. A decrease in coronary tone or relief of spasm may also be of importance. Therefore, if clinical tolerance is a real phenomenon, it is not clearly understood which basic action(s) of nitrates are affected, or if all are involved.

Another unknown question relates to whether one nitrate formulation has a greater potential to induce tolerance than another. Needleman's rat experiments suggest this, indicating that ISDN may be the least tolerance-producing nitrate tested in vitro (6, 7). Further work in this area is clearly needed.

Conclusions

1. Nitroglycerin tolerance is a real phenomenon. Old and new evidence attests to this, although the clinical significance remains controversial. Industrial experience in the explosives- and nitroglycerin-manufacturing industries has amply demonstrated the danger of abruptly stopping nitrate exposure (4, 37); if tolerance to nitrates was complete, there would appear to be no explanation for "withdrawal" vasoconstriction and coronary vasospasm (Monday headache, chest pain syndromes).
2. Reflex or counterregulatory adaptive mechanisms that come into play during chronic nitrate administration are probably very important but are inadequately characterized. The role of the autonomic nervous system, catecholamine synthesis and release, etc., are unknown. Clearly, important vasoregulatory alterations occur in any subject given potent vasodilators. Some have stressed that the decreased or totally absent blood pressure and heart rate responses following chronic

20

nitrate therapy may really represent "pseudotolerance", as the integrated response of the circulatory system and central nervous system come into play to "protect" against nitrate-induced hypotension.

3. The precise mechanism(s) for tolerance are poorly understood. Future work assessing nitrate blood vessel receptors and nitroglycerin tissue kinetics holds potential promise in elucidating this complex subject. Altered metabolism or excretion of parent nitrate does not appear to play a major role in the development of tolerance.

4. From a clinician's perspective it is reasonable to conclude that the wealth of observations in thousands of patients treated with nitrates and the large number of negative studies on nitrate tolerance indicate that tolerance is not a common or important problem in everyday practice. Long-acting nitrates appear to be bioavailable and physiologically effective in most patients with angina and congestive heart failure after weeks, months, or even years of treatment.

5. Scattered reports continue to appear suggesting that tolerance can develop in subjects given nitrates. The well-known loss of nitrate headaches during chronic treatment, as well as the repeatedly documented attenuation of nitrate-induced decreases in blood pressure and increases in heart rate, support this view. In some or perhaps most instances, these hemodynamic alterations may relate to chronic circulatory adjustments that occur with the chronic use of vasodilators. This may result in pseudotolerance with maintained effectiveness of clinical endpoints (e.g., increased exercise duration and decreased ischemia in angina, decreased left-ventricular filling pressure in chronic congestive heart failure). The best evidence supporting nitrate tolerance comes from the study of Thadani et al. (12–14), and even here the clinical effects of ISDN with respect to antianginal protection were reduced only in respect of duration of protection but not in respect of the degree of protection.

6. Dose-response relationships during chronic treatment have been inadequately investigated. Evidence suggests that once sustained levels of nitrates and metabolites are present in the plasma (perhaps indirectly reflecting the degree of receptor binding and tissue saturation), the enhanced physiological response to increasing amounts of nitrate readily demonstrable in acute dosing studies may disappear.

7. It has been suggested that transitory interruption of nitrate therapy for a period as short as several hours may enhance continuing responsiveness to nitrates. Most, but not all, studies not supportive of tolerance employ a nitrate-free interval of 6 or more hours before the challenge nitrate dose is given. Much more work is needed to resolve this point. If this is true, current efforts to provide sustained therapeutic nitroglycerin levels over a 24-h-period may be misguided, as tolerance could be more readily induced by such therapy.

8. Nitrate therapy should always be administered intelligently. Dosage should be increased carefully to a clinical endpoint (e.g., angina improvement, decrease in "backward failure"). Side-effects, particularly headaches, dizziness, and orthostatic symptoms, can usually be controlled by patient counseling, reducing the dosage for several days, or waiting for the typical disappearance of these side-effects. It must be recognized that occasional patients do not respond to nitrates, whereas others are exquisitely sensitive. Always use the lowest effective dose but be prepared to employ very high dosages in the unusual patient who fails to respond to more conventional dosing. Never abruptly taper long-acting nitrate therapy in patients with underlying coronary disease. When symptoms increase in a patient on chronic nitrate therapy, carefully reevaluate the clinical setting. The clinical deterioration may be a result of progression of native disease, exacerbating factors, true nitrate tolerance, or patient noncompliance. Fortunately, loss of symptom relief during nitrate therapy is relatively uncommon in clinical practice, an observation that definitely militates against nitrate tolerance as a common or important problem.

References

1. Abrams J: Oral long acting nitrates in angina pectoris and the rationale for high dose therapy. Brit J Clin Practice Suppl 12, pp. 39–43, 1981.
2. Shane SJ: High dose oral isosorbide dinitrate and ischemic heart pain. Can Fam Phys 19: 61–65 (1973).
3. Stewart DD: Remarkable tolerance to nitroglycerin. Philadelphia Polyclinic. p. 172.
4. Abrams J: Nitrate tolerance and dependence. Amer Heart J 99: 113–123 (1980).

5. Abrams J: Nitrate tolerance and dependence. A critical assessment. La Nouv Presse Médic 9: 2499–2504 (1980).

6. Needleman P, Johnson EM: The pharmacological and biochemical interaction of organic nitrates with sulfhydryls: possible correlations with the mechanism for tolerance development, vasodilation and mitochondrial and enzyme reactions, in Needleman P. ed: Handbook of Experimental Pharmacology, New York, 1975, Springer-Verlag, Inc., V. 40, pp. 97–114.

7. Needleman P, Johnson EM: Mechanism of tolerance development to organic nitrates, J Pharmacol Exp Ther 184: 709 (1973).

8. Crandall LA et al.: Acquired tolerance to and cross tolerance between the nitrous and nitric acid esters and sodium nitrite in man. J Pharmacol Exp Ther 41: 103 (1931).

9. Schelling J, Lasagna L: A study of cross-tolerance to circulatory effects of organic nitrates. Clin Pharmacol Ther 8: 256–260 (1966).

10. Zelis R, Mason DT: Isosorbide dinitrate. Effect on the vasodilation response to nitroglycerin. JAMA 234: 166–169 (1975).

11. Needleman P: Tolerance to the vascular effects of glyceryl trinitrate. J Pharmacol Exper Ther 171: 990–102 (1970).

12. Thadani U, Fung H, Darke AC, Parker JO: Oral isosorbide dinitrate in the treatment of angina pectoris. Dose-response relationship and duration of action during acute therapy. Circulation 62: 491–502 (1980).

13. Thadani U, Manyari D, Parker JO, Fung H: Tolerance to the circulatory effects of oral isosorbide dinitrate. Rate of development and cross-tolerance to glyceryl trinitrate. Circulation 61: 526–535 (1980).

14. Thadani U, Fung H, Darke AC, Parker JO: Oral isosorbide dinitrate in angina pectoris. Comparison of duration of action and dose response relationship during acute and sustained therapy. Amer J Cardiol 49: 411 (1982).

15. Lee G, Mason DT, DeMaria A: Effects of long-term oral administration of isosorbide dinitrate on the antianginal response to nitroglycerin. Absence of cross-tolerance and self-tolerance shown by exercise testing. Am J Cardiol 41: 82–87 (1978.

16. Danahy DT, Aronow WS: Hemodynamics and antianginal effects of high dose oral isosorbide dinitrate after chronic use. Circulation 56: 205–212 (1977).

17. Abrams J: Usefulness of long-acting nitrates in cardiovascular disease. Am J Med 64: 103–104 (1978).

18a. Rudolph W, Blasini R, Froer KL et al.: Effects of acute and chronic administration of isosorbide dinitrat, sustained-release form, in patients with angina pectoris. In Lichtlen et al., eds.: Nitrates III, Berlin, 1981 Springer-Verlag, pp. 75–81.

18b. Blasini R, Brügmann U, Manns A, Froer KL, Hall D, Rudolph W: Wirksamkeit von Isosorbiddinitrat in retardierter Form bei Langzeitbehandlung; Herz 5: 298–305 (1980).

19. Lee G, Mason DT, Amsterdam EA et al.: Antianginal efficacy of oral therapy with isosorbide dinitrate capsules. Chest 73: 327 (1978).

20. Tauchert M, Jansen W, Osterspey A, Fuchs M, Hombach V, Hilger HH: Hemodynamic effects of 5-isosorbide mononitrate during acute and chronic administration. This volume p. 43.

21. Franciosa JA, Cohn JN: Sustained hemodynamic effects without tolerance during long-term isosorbide dinitrate treatment in chronic left ventricular failure. Am J Cardiol 45: 640–654 (1980).

22. Becker HJ, Walden G, Kaltenbach M: Gibt es eine „Tachyphylaxie" bzw. eine Gewöhnung bei der Behandlung der Angina pectoris und Nitroglycerin. Verh Dt Ges Inn Med 82, 1208–1210 (1976).

23. Becker HJ et al. 1980 (personal communication).

24. Becker H-J, Mendt R, Kretschmer S, Hüwer HD: Tolerance in Patients with Coronary Heart Disease Under Chronic Treatment with Isosorbide Dinitrate? This volume p. 117.

25. Schneider W et al.: Long-term effects of high-dose ISDN therapy in patients with coronary heart disease. This volume p. 131.

26. Distante A, L'Abbate A, Palombo C et al: May Prolonged high doses of nitrates cause tolerance? Preliminary results on the response to an additional dose by infusion. In Lichtlen PR et al, eds.: Nitrates III, Berlin, 1981, Springer-Verlag, pp. 82–90.

27. Brunner D, Weisbord J, Meshulam N, Margulis S: Unchanged efficacy of acute sublingual nitrate compounds during long-term treatment with percutaneously applied isosorbide dinitrate ointment. In Lichtlen PR et al, eds: Nitrates III, Berlin, 1981, Springer-Verlag, pp. 100–109.

28. Distante A, Moscarelli E, Morales MA et al: Chronic treatment of ischemic heart disease with isosorbide dinitrate retard tablets: evidence of preserved hemodynamic response to a sublingual dose of 5 mg. This volume p. 161.
29. Niederer W et al.: Hemodynamic and ventricular dynamic investigations of nitrate tolerance. This volume p. 65.
30. Hauf GF, Bubenheimer P, Roskamm H: Treatment of congestive heart failure with vasodilators. Comparison of acute and long-term effects of various drug classes. This volume p. 77.
31. Bassan M, Weiler-Ravell D, The additive antianginal action of oral isosorbide dinitrate in patients receiving propranolol: and duration of effect. Personal communication
32. Armstrong-Moffat JA, Marks GS, Armstrong PW: Effects of Sustained nitroglycerin delivery on the arterial venous gradient in the dog. Clin and Invest Med 4: 7B (1981).
33. Armstrong-Moffat JA, Marks GS, Watts DG, Armstrong PW: Tolerance to the hemodynamic effects of nitroglycerin. Canad Cardiovas Soc, Montreal, Oct. 1981 (abstr.).
34. Fung HL: Pharmacokinetics of isosorbide dinitrate during tolerance development. This volume p. 25.
35. Fung HL, Kamiya A: Disposition of nitroglycerin in rat plasma and selected blood vessels. Intern Congress of Pharmacol, Tokyo, July, 1981 (abstr).
36. Becker LC, Fortuin NJ, Pitt B: Effect of ischemia and antianginal drugs on the distribution of radioactive microspheres on the canine left ventricle. Circulation Res 28: 263–269 (1971).
37. Lange RL, Reid MS, Tresch DD et al: Non-atheromatous ischemic heart disease following withdrawal from chronic industrial nitroglycerin exposure. Circulation 46: 666 (1972).

Author's address:
Jonathan Abrams
Professor of Medicine
Chief, Division of Cardiology
Department of Medicine
University of New Mexico School of Medicine
Albuquerque, New Mexico 87131

Pharmacokinetics of Isosorbide Dinitrate During Tolerance Development

Ho-Leung Fung

One of the central questions posed in this symposium is: "Does chronic use of organic nitrates in the clinical setting lead to tolerance of their beneficial effects?" The various chapters address the clinical evidence for and against this hypothesis. The purpose of the present discussion is, however, to examine whether chronic nitrate dosing produces changes in its pharmacokinetics, i.e., in the rates and extents of absorption, distribution, and elimination of the drug in the body, and to determine whether these pharmacokinetic changes, if present, are consistent with the various mechanisms that can be proposed for nitrate tolerance.

There has only been a small number of pharmacokinetic studies that relate particularly to this issue. In a protocol that our group at Buffalo carried out jointly with Thadani and Parker at Kingston (Canada), we examined the circulatory and exercise parameters, as well as the pharmacokinetics of isosorbide dinitrate (ISDN), after single and chronic dosing in 12 angina patients. Details of this study have been presented elsewhere (1–3). In brief, the conclusions reached were that chronic oral dosing for 1 week, with doses of 15, 30, 60, or 120 mg ISDN four times daily, led to significant diminution in the intensity and duration of changes in heart rate, blood pressure, and exercise tolerance. In these patients, plasma ISDN concentrations were shown to increase, rather than decrease, after chronic dosing. This observation would clearly be inconsistent with any hypothesis of ISDN tolerance that might involve enhanced systemic metabolism of this organic nitrate.

This conclusion also appears to be applicable to nitroglycerin, on the basis of data available on its pharmacokinetics in relation to tolerance development. Thadani et al. (4) showed that plasma nitroglycerin concentrations resulting from sublingual dosing were essentially unaffected after development of cross-tolerance to ISDN given orally. Armstrong-Moffat et al. (5) recently studied the dose-response relationship for intravenous nitroglycerin in anesthetized dogs before and after administration of nitroglycerin ointment (36 mg every 8 h for 5 days). These investigators found a significant reduction in the observed systolic blood pressure after ointment application. The diminution in hemodynamic response was observed in spite of higher plasma nitroglycerin concentrations at the second trial.

These data showed that nitrate tolerance is accompanied either by little change or by an increase in plasma nitrate concentration. A conclusion that may possibly be drawn is that plasma nitrate concentration is irrelevant in the examination of the tolerance phenomenon. Alternatively, it may be suggested that the relationship between plasma concentration and tolerance is complex and multifactorial, and that its elucidation requires a clearer understanding of the intermediate parameters and processes linking these two variables.

For the latter purpose, it might be useful to view nitrate action from a pharmacokinetic perspective. Figure 1 shows a scheme that attempts to bring into focus the interplay between nitrate pharmacokinetics and pharmacodynamics. Plasma nitrate concentration is

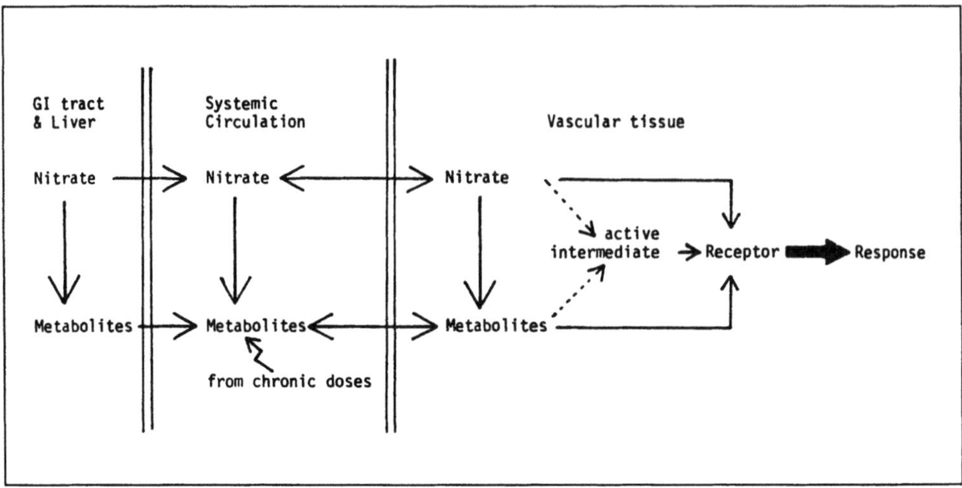

Fig. 1. Schematization of nitrate action from a pharmacokinetic viewpoint. *GI,* gastrointestinal.

controlled by a number of processes, among which are input (absorption and first-pass metabolism), systemic metabolism, and distribution to peripheral tissues. It is assumed, perhaps not unreasonably, that the principal site of nitrate action is in (or on) the vascular tissue. Fung and Kamiya (6) have shown that vascular uptake of nitroglycerin is extensive, and may be site- and/or concentration-dependent. Thus plasma nitrate concentration can be viewed as a determinant (a driving force), or in other cases as a reflection (see later), of the extent of drug distribution into this presumed receptor phase. Once this distribution has taken place, nitrate in the vascular tissue can elicit a response by either reacting with the receptor directly, or through an active intermediate. The latter pathway, involving S-nitrosothiols, has recently been demonstrated by Ignarro et al. (7).

From the scheme proposed (Fig. 1), it appears possible that nitrate tolerance can be effected through a number of independent or coexisting mechanisms, each of which may produce a different set of pharmacokinetic consequences. The classical model proposed by Needleman and associates (8) suggested that tolerance is caused by a depletion of reduced sulfhydryl groups at the receptor site. With this biochemical model, the pertinent pharmacokinetic species to examine is that of free sulfhydryl. Among the positive evidence for this model are that dithiothreitol, a potent thiol, reverses nitroglycerin tolerance and that ethacrynic acid, a thiol aklylating agent, decreases vascular responsiveness (8). Keith and Burkman (9) showed recently, however, that maximal tolerance to nitroglycerin occurs prior to any detectable decrease in tissue sulfhydryl content. The Needleman sulfhydryl model of nitrate tolerance is therefore inconsistent with this finding.

Another possible model that may be suggested is one that involves reduced availability or activity of the active intermediate (i.e., S-nitrosothiol) during the tolerant state. This might be brought about by reduced formation or accelerated decomposition of the active intermediate, or through inhibited interaction with the receptor(s). Reduced formation of the active intermediate can be caused by a reduction in the available pool of free thiols (a mechanism essentially compatible with Needleman's hypothesis), and/or by a reduction in the nitrate concentration in the vascular tissue. In this model, the pertinent pharmaco-

26

kinetic analysis should be that of the active intermediate. Unfortunately, no information is available at this time regarding the fate and kinetics of the presumed intermediate during tolerance development.

Yet a third possible mechanism of nitrate tolerance can be proposed. This model is similar to one aspect of the second suggested mechanism in that tolerance might have been brought about by decreased concentration of unchanged nitrate in the vascular tissue. This model, however, does not require nitrate action to be mediated via an active intermediate (i.e., nitrate interacts with the receptor directly). Thus, according to this mechanism, nitrate pharmacokinetics during tolerance might be sufficiently altered for distribution into the vascular tissue to be reduced, for example. Here, the pharmacokinetic consequence might be reflected in the plasma nitrate concentration: with decreased distribution into the peripheral tissue, a smaller apparent volume of distribution and thus also higher plasma concentrations are observed. The experimental observation of higher ISDN levels after chronic dosing in humans (2) may then be consistent with this model. Animal studies in my laboratory (10) have shown that both metabolites of ISDN, the 2- and 5-mononitrates of isosorbide, significantly reduced the apparent volume of distribution of ISDN. These metabolites may be accumulated during chronic dosing and could thus possibly play a role in tolerance development. Experimental studies are now in process to examine whether tolerance development might alter the uptake and/or disposition of nitrate in vascular tissue.

In summary, the available data on plasma nitrate kinetics do not offer a direct or simple explanation of nitrate tolerance. This phenomenon might be better understood, however, if pharmacokinetic determinations on nitrates, and possibly their active intermediates, are carried out in the presumed site of pharmacological action, namely the vascular tissue (6).

Acknowledgement: Supported in part by NIH grant HL22273.

References

1. Thadani U, Fung H-L, Darke AC, and Parker JO, "Oral Isosorbide Dinitrate in the Treatment of Angina Pectoris. Dose Response Relationship and Duration of Action During Acute Therapy", Circulation 62: 491–502 (1980).

2. Fung H-L, McNiff EF, Ruggirello D, Darke A, Thadani U, and Parker JO, "Kinetics of Isosorbide Dinitrate and Relationships to Pharmacological Effects", Brit J Clin Pharmacol 11: 579–590 (1981).

3. Thadani U, Fung H-L, Darke AC, and Parker JO, "Oral Isosorbide Dinitrate in Angina Pectoris. Comparison of Duration of Action and Dose Response Relationship during Acute and Sustained Therapy", Am J Cardiol, in press.

4. Thadani U, Manyari D, Parker JO, and Fung H-L, "Tolerance to the Circulatory Effects of Oral Isosorbide Dinitrate. Rate of Development and Cross Tolerance to Glyceryl Trinitrate", Circulation 61: 526–535 (1980).

5. Armstrong-Moffat JA, Marks GS, Watts DG, and Armstrong PW, "Tolerance to the Hemodynamic Effects of Nitroglycerin", Abstract of the Scientific Program, the 34th Annual Meeting of the Canadian Cardiovascular Society, October 28–31, 1981, p. 111.

6. Fung H-L, and Kamiya A, "Disposition of Nitroglycerin in Rat Plasma and Selected Blood Vessels", Abstracts of the Eighth International Congress of Pharmacology, July 19–24, 1981, Tokyo, p. 552.

7. Ignarro LJ, Lippton H, Edwards JC, Baricos WH, Hyman AL, Kadowitz PJ, and Gruetter CA, "Mechanism of Vascular Smooth Muscle Relaxation by Organic Nitrates, Nitrites, Nitroprusside, and Nitric Oxide: Evidence for the Involvement of S-Nitrosothiols as Active Intermediates", J Pharmacol Exp Ther 218: 739–749 (1981).
8. Needleman P, Jakschik B, and Johnson EM, "Sulfhydryl Requirement for Relaxation of Vascular Smooth Muscle", J Pharmacol Exp Ther 187: 324–331 (1973).
9. Keith RA, and Burkman AM, "In Vitro Induction of Nitroglycerin (NTG) Tolerance in Vascular Tissue at pH 7.4 and 9.0 Occurs Prior to the Decrease in Sulfhydryl (SH) Content", Fed Proc (abstract) 40: 729 (1981).
10. Morrison RA, and Fung H-L, unpublished data.

Author's address:
Ho-Leung Fung
Department of Pharmaceutics,
School of Pharmacy
State University of New York at Buffalo,
Amherst, NY, 14260 USA

Discussion

GLEICHMANN:

I have a question to Dr. Abrams regarding connections between systolic blood pressure and tolerance. We have heard this morning from Dr. Schneider that during long-term therapy with high doses of ISDN, one or two patients out of fifteen had developed hypotension which was classified as an untoward effect. Do you think that these were patients without tolerance and all the others developed tolerance? This would fit into the concept that tolerance may develop in the arterial bed, but not in the venous system.

ABRAMS:

I don't think I can answer that with any certainty. All of the studies show individual variability and although we are looking at, and talking about, group responses, there are always patients or individuals who have an excessive or a very blunt response, again as anyone who has carried out nitrate research knows that there are some individuals who do not respond at all to acute administration of isosorbide dinitrate or nitroglycerin or who at least have a very minimal response and others have an excessive one. I think that everyone who has a marked vascular response after chronic dosing clearly has not developed tolerance. The group from Pisa holds that nitrates mainly act upon the coronary artery system. Most of the other groups believe that the peripheral effect on the venous bed are more important. Probably the mechanisms of nitrates in angina pectoris are complex and involve vasomotor tone, coronary tone as well as pre- and afterload reduction.

FRANCIOSA:

I have a question to Dr. Fung. I am going to raise the issue again of apparent tolerance and real tolerance. I am still bothered by using blood pressure, angina and so forth as an indicator of tolerance, because any vasodilator, of course, will produce reflex stimulation in the sympathetic nervous system, which can certainly upset blood pressure, aggravate angina, change ST-segment, and we call this apparent tolerance. Do you have any data directly looking at circulating catecholamine levels in your studies , and is there any information about what catecholamines do to the so-called nitrate receptor?

FUNG:

We did not determine catecholamine concentrations and I don't know about results of other investigations in man. There is some evidence of the effects of nitrates on catecholamines in animals. Nitrates can also influence prostaglandines. We have given nitroglycerin intravenously and have investigated the influence on platelet aggregation and measured at the same time prostaglandine concentration in plasma. We saw no change in prostacycline concentration, but this is not to say that there is none. These measurements are very difficult, as are catecholamine determinationes.

WOODCOCK:

I would like to make a comment to the finding by Dr. Fung that the maximum response, produced by long-term treatment with different doses of isosorbide dinitrate, from 15 to 120 mg, consisted in the same drop in blood pressure. This finding, to my mind, tells us that there is not a change in the number of receptors, but rather a change in the nature of the receptors and maybe a change from perhaps a mixture of high and low affinity to all high-affinity receptors. A change in the number or a loss of low affinity receptors could be due to the presence of 5-mononitrate or 2-mononitrate, and Dr. Fung has shown us that the 5-, or the 2-mononitrate can interfere with the distribution of isosorbide dinitrate. This could explain this form of tolerance on a molecular basis.

FUNG:

Certainly that is one way to look at the problem. But it may be interpreted that we had reached the plateau of the response curve, and therefore after chronic dosing the number of receptors is constant, regardless of the drug concentration. Maybe we should investigate the intermediate products, which are very unstable. They could not yet been measured in vitro, but it should be possible to synthesize them and determine their vasodilating activity.

KALTENBACH:

Dr. Fung, you mentioned that one problem in your study may be the non-randomization of dosage. In our study, it was randomized. There might be another problem, that the placebo period always followed the acute period. And then you compared the results of this placebo experiment with those at the end of a long-term treatment without using a placebo period at the end of the long-term treatment.

DEMARIA:

I wonder if anyone on the panel would want to comment on how the pharmacodynamics might relate to the alleged differences in vascular responsiveness, say between the cerebral circulation and the peripheral vascular circulation? If we accept the difference in tolerance to headaches and what was alleged to be tolerance to antianginal effects, and for instance if we go back and look at Zelis's study where he showed that venous tone manifested tolerance whereas arteriolar tone did not, how would that fit into these pharmacodynamic theories of receptors, etc.?

FUNG:

Perhaps I can answer somewhat indirectly. We had measured the uptake of nitroglycerin by large venous vessels and large arterial vessels. If we express the data in nanograms of nitroglycerin per gram of vessel wall, there appears to be a more intensive uptake of nitrates into the venous vessels than into the aorta. However, I hasten to add that we are measuring the whole vessel wall and not quantity of substance per gram of receptor. This has to be pointed out because the vascular structures are very different. Perhaps we ought to use cultures of arterial and venous cells to examine it on a cellular basis.

ABRAMS:

There was a study from the United States a few years ago showing a different responsiveness of large and small coronary vessels. There are also results from Switzerland (P. Imhof in Nitrates III*) which suggest that nitrate effects on the venous system occur at lower dosages than on the arterial system. Treating patients with heart failure, reduction of left ventricular diameters is only seen with higher nitrate doses. These studies have nothing in particular to do with tolerance, but show the bias of using different doses in different studies.

FRANCIOSA:

I think it is important to not just consider the different vessels but also the different nitrates we are talking about. Dr. Needleman has shown on the sulfhydryl model that the various nitrates behave differently.

---

* Editor's note

30

FUNG:

Because we had this pharmacokinetic observation in humans we wanted to reproduce it in animals, in rats primarily, and we have been trying for 6 months to induce vascular tolerance with the Needleman aortic strip model. We couldn't induce it with maximal doses of ISDN, but it occurred with very small doses of nitroglycerin.

BECKER:

I would like to make a comment from a clinician's point of view. When patients were losing their headaches during nitrate treatment this has been regarded as a partial tolerance. The disappearance of headaches could, however, be the result of adaptation to vasodilation. The mentioned problem of nitrate withdrawal is a very good argument against tolerance, as is the advice to avoid abrupt discontinuation of nitrate therapy.

ABRAMS:

To my knowledge, neither the withdrawal syndrome nor dependence were re-assessed by clinical studies. No one has looked at this in angina patients. Dr. Franciosa suggested in a paper a couple of years ago, based on really anecdotal and small numbers of patients that withdrawal may be a problem, especially with nitroprusside and other vasodilators. He indicated that abrupt cessation may not be good. I really feel that one should carefully take a patient off high dose long-acting nitrates. In summary, I think tolerance is not a big problem.

BUSSMANN:

Dr. Fung, in the study together with Thadani, you found a steep fall in systolic blood pressure in the standing position down to 80 mm Hg. Yet, even in this acute study, you did not find a clear dose-response relation since the 60 mg dose caused the lowest blood pressure, instead of the 120 mg dose. You found a large difference between acute and chronic effects which seems to indicate tolerance to this hemodynamic effect. One should, however, bear in mind that systolic blood pressure cannot be reduced to 80 mm Hg after each dose continuously. This will be counter-regulated. So I think this phenomenon is nothing else than pseudo-tolerance based on counterregulation.

FUNG:

The compensatory effect is a very important factor in relating dose-response or concentration-response to nitrates. While a single dose did produce a large change, when we were titrating it from 15 mg four times a day up to 120 mg four times a day, there was a gradual adaptation. It is more a semantic problem, how to call diminution of response. The walking time also seems to be an issue of discussion as to its validity as a method of measurement; the walking time had also shown statistical differences under acute dosing at 8 hours at all doses, whereas there was no statistical difference in walking time after 4, 6, and 8 hours with chronic doses of isosorbide dinitrate.

Lack of Tolerance Development to the Hemodynamic Effects of Nitrates in Patients with Chronic Congestive Heart Failure

Joseph A. Franciosa

Introduction

The beneficial acute hemodynamic effects of vasodilators in patients with congestive heart failure are well established (1, 2). The use of vasodilators in long-term management of chronic heart failure is being intensively evaluated, and nitrates are among the earliest and most extensively studied agents employed for chronic afterload reduction (3–7). Loss of hemodynamic efficacy of some vasodilators has been demonstrated in patients with heart failure, while tolerance to nitrates as antianginal agents has been suggested (8–10). Furthermore, the venodilating effect of nitrates may become blunted with time (11). It is therefore extremely important to establish long-term hemodynamic efficacy of nitrates if they are to be important in the treatment of chronic congestive heart failure.

Nitrate Effects on Resting Hemodynamics in Heart Failure

Nitrates improve resting hemodynamics in patients with left-ventricular failure by decreasing left-ventricular filling pressure and usually raising cardiac output (2, 4, 5, 7). Schelling and Lasagna showed that long-acting nitrates can attenuate the blood-pressure-lowering effect of nitroglycerin (10). However, changes in systemic arterial pressure may not be a reliable indicator of nitrate effects, since blood pressure regulation is complex and compensatory mechanisms are triggered by a sudden fall in blood pressure. Furthermore, nitrates tend to be more potent venodilators than arterial dilators. We have therefore studied the question of nitrate tolerance in patients with heart failure, utilizing changes in pulmonary wedge pressure as a measure of responsiveness (12).

Studies were performed in 19 patients with chronic left-ventricular failure due to ischemic or idiopathic cardiomyopathy. All patients were receiving maintenance digitalis and diuretic therapy for symptoms of congestive heart failure that had been present for at least 3 months. All patients had clinical and radiological evidence of congestive heart failure with an average cardiothoracic ratio of $57 \pm 5\%$ (SD). Patients with recent myocardial infarction, angina pectoris, primary valvular heart disease, or primary lung disease were excluded.

Swan-Ganz catheterization was performed for measurement of pulmonary arterial pressures, and cardiac output was measured by the carbon dioxide rebreathing method which we have previously validated in patients with heart failure (13, 14). Heart rate and rhythm were recorded from the electrocardiogram and blood pressure was measured by the standard cuff technique.

On the first day of study control hemodynamic measurements were obtained at supine rest, after which isosorbide dinitrate (ISDN), 40 mg orally, was administered. Measurements were repeated 90 min later. All patients were given active drug on day 1 to assure that all responded to the nitrate. After completing day 1 studies, patients were randomly assigned in double-blind fashion to receive 40 mg ISDN four times daily or placebo tablets four times daily. This regimen, along with digitalis and diuretics, was continued for 3 months. At the end of 3 months patients were instructed to withhold diuretics for 24 h before reporting to the laboratory, where they were given all their usual medications except for the test drug and diuretics. Swan-Ganz catheterization was again performed and all measurements repeated as on day 1 before and 90 min after administration of the coded test drug. Of the 19 patients who completed the trial, ten received placebo and nine ISDN.

Characteristics of the patient populations are summarized in Table 1. The groups were similar in age, cause and severity of heart failure, heart size, and hemodynamics, which showed increased pulmonary wedge pressure with reduced cardiac index.

Table 1. Baseline characteristics of patients with congestive heart failure

	Isosorbide dinitrate	Placebo
Number of patients	9	10
Age (years)	57 ± 7	59 ± 6
Etiology of heart failure		
Ischemic cardiomyopathy	5	7
Idiopathic cardiomyopathy	4	3
Clinical class*	2.8 ± 0.7	3 ± 0.5
Cardiothoracic ratio (%)	56 ± 6	58 ± 3
Pulmonary wedge pressure (mmHg)	26 ± 8	24 ± 8
Cardiac index ($l/min/m^2$)	2.1 ± 0.8	2.1 ± 0.6

Values = mean and SD; no differences are statistically significant.
* According to criteria of the New York Heart Association.

Table 2. Hemodynamic effects of long-term isosorbide dinitrate administration to patients with chronic congestive heart failure

	Isosorbide dinitrate		Placebo	
	Control	Treated 3 months	Control	Treated 3 months
Heart rate (beats/min)	82 ± 11	82 ± 14	82 ± 11	89 ± 14
Mean arterial pressure (mmHg)	91 ± 13	97 ± 7	85 ± 9	91 ± 8
Pulmonary wedge pressure (mmHg)	26 ± 8	23 ± 3*	24 ± 8	23 ± 7
Cardiac index ($l/min/m^2$)	2.1 ± 0.8	2.1 ± 0.9	2.1 ± 0.6	1.9 ± 0.8
Systemic vascular resistance (units)	25 ± 7	27 ± 10	23 ± 6	29 ± 15

Values = mean and standard deviation; no differences in control values between groups are significant; * $p < 0.02$ compared to control

Hemodynamic responses to the first dose of ISDN were similar in both groups. Pulmonary wedge pressure fell from 26 ± 8 to 18 ± 5 mmHg in the group assigned to ISDN, while in those later given placebo, pulmonary wedge pressure fell from 24 ± 8 to 14 ± 6 mmHg (both $p < 0.001$). Mean arterial blood pressure also fell significantly in both groups after the initial dose of ISDN, while other hemodynamic changes were not significant in either group. Thus both groups of patients were similarly responsive to ISDN.

After 3 months of placebo treatment, resting hemodynamics were not different from control (Table 2). In those patients treated with ISDN, however, after 3 months the pulmonary wedge pressure was still modestly but significantly reduced from control (Table 2). It must be recalled that measurements at 3 months were made at least 8 h from the last previous dose of test drug, a time interval which exceeds the known duration of effect of single doses of ISDN (4).

Table 3. Hemodynamic responses to single doses of isosorbide dinitrate (ISDN) at control and after 3 months of treatment

	Percentage change after		
	First dose ISDN	Single dose ISDN after 3 months	Single dose placebo after 3 months
Heart rate	− 2	8	−4
Mean arterial pressure	− 6*	−10**	−1
Pulmonary wedge pressure	−31***	−23**	−6
Cardiac index	5	31	7

$* p < 0.05; ** p < 0.01; *** p < 0.001$

The effects of single doses of test drug given after 3 months of their continuous administration are summarized in Table 3. In patients receiving ISDN, a single dose of this agent after 3 months produced significant reductions in mean arterial pressure and pulmonary wedge pressure similar to the effects seen when the first dose of nitrate was given 3 months earlier. Cardiac index also tended to increase more after a single dose of nitrate at 3 months, but the change was not statistically significant due to marked variability in individual responses. Placebo administration after 3 months of placebo treatment had no significant hemodynamic effects. Thus we observed no evidence of development of tolerance to the hemodynamic effects of ISDN during its long-term administration to patients with chronic left-ventricular failure.

Since our patients all received diuretics during the treatment period, data were analyzed to see if this influenced responses to ISDN. In four patients treated with nitrate, diuretic dosage had been increased, but their fall in pulmonary wedge pressure after a single dose of ISDN at 3 months averaged 3 ± 1 mmHg, which was not different from the 5 ± 2 mmHg fall observed in patients whose diuretics were unchanged. Likewise, responses in placebo-treated patients were also uninfluenced by changes in diuretic dosage.

Nitrate Effects on Exercise Hemodynamics in Heart Failure

Heart failure symptoms are usually precipitated or worsened by exertion. Furthermore, resting hemodynamics may not reliably reflect exercise hemodynamics (15). We have therefore also observed the effects of ISDN on exercise hemodynamics and exercise capacity in patients with congestive heart failure.

Hemodynamic measurements were also made during upright bicycle exercise in 17 of the 19 patients enrolled in the present study. The exercise protocol and a detailed report of the results of these exercise studies have been reported elsewhere (16, 17). We are presently reporting only the hemodynamic responses to single doses of ISDN at control and after 3 months of nitrate treatment:

Table 4. Effects of isosorbide dinitrate on exercise hemodynamics in patients with chronic congestive heart failure

	Isosorbide dinitrate		Placebo	
	Change after first dose$^\circ$	Change after single dose after 3 months	Change after first dose$^\circ$	Change after single dose after 3 months
Mean arterial pressure (mmHg)	-3 ± 6	-1 ± 6	-8 ± 13	0 ± 12
Pulmonary wedge pressure (mmHg)	$-7 \pm 5^{**}$	$-5 \pm 2^{**}$	$-7 \pm 9^{*}$	2 ± 7

Values = mean and standard deviation
$^\circ$ First dose was isosorbide dinitrate in both groups
* $p < 0.05$; ** $p < 0.01$

The results are summarized in Table 4. The first dose of ISDN had no significant effect on mean arterial pressure during exercise, but pulmonary wedge pressure was significantly reduced after the first dose of nitrate. The magnitude of reduction in pulmonary wedge pressure during exercise was similar in patients ultimately given long-term treatment with ISDN or placebo. After 3 months of continuous therapy, a single dose of ISDN still lowered pulmonary wedge pressure significantly during exercise, and the response was similar to that observed after the initial dose 3 months earlier. In the placebo-treated group there were no significant hemodynamic responses noted at 3 months before or after a single dose of placebo. Since these patients were also responsive to nitrates initially, the results cannot be explained by differences in patient populations. Neither ISDN nor placebo produced any significant changes in heart rate, cardiac index, stroke volume, or systemic vascular resistance during exercise.

The significance of these nitrate-induced changes in exercise hemodynamics is not clear, since exercise duration and maximal oxygen uptake in these patients increased significantly after 3 months but not after the first dose, despite similar hemodynamic responses to ISDN each time (17).

38

Conclusions

The present results demonstrate that the hemodynamic effects of large oral doses of ISDN both at rest and during exercise are sustained without the development of tolerance during their long-term administration in patients with chronic left-ventricular failure. The present studies employed pulmonary wedge pressure, which is a sensitive indicator of responsiveness to nitrates. Previous reports of nitrate tolerance may relate to the use of less specific and sensitive indicators, such as systemic arterial blood pressure. On the basis of our results, hemodynamic tolerance to nitrates does not appear to be an important problem associated with their use in treating chronic congestive heart failure. Nevertheless, some form of nitrate tolerance may indeed exist, since the clinical occurrence of headaches decreases in frequency and intensity with continued nitrate administration in patients with angina pectoris or heart failure (6, 12, 18). Finally, the importance of the demonstration of sustained hemodynamic efficacy of nitrates should not be overemphasized, since hemodynamic improvement may not correlate with symptomatic improvement (19, 20). Proof of efficacy of vasodilators in the treatment of chronic left-ventricular failure requires demonstration of beneficial effects on morbidity and mortality in properly designed and controlled trials. Improved hemodynamics and exercise capacity, while desirable and encouraging, nevertheless do not represent the ultimate goal of therapy.

References

1. Cohn JN, Franciosa JA: Drug therapy: vasodilator therapy of cardiac failure. N Engl J Med 297: 27 and 254 (1977).
2. Franciosa JA, Cohn JN: Hemodynamic responsiveness to short- and long-acting vasodilators in left ventricular failure. Am J Med 65: 126 (1978).
3. Mason DT: Vasodilator and inotropic therapy of heart failure: symposium perspective. Am J Med 65: 101 (1978).
4. Franciosa JA, Mikulic E, Cohn JN, Jose E, Fabie A: Hemodynamic effects of orally administered isosorbide dinitrate in patients with congestive heart failure. Circulation 50: 1020 (1974).
5. Franciosa JA, Blank RC, Cohn JN: Nitrate effects on cardiac output and left ventricular outflow resistance in chronic congestive heart failure. Am J Med 64: 207 (1978).
6. Franciosa JA, Nordstrom LA, Cohn JN: Nitrate therapy for congestive heart failure. JAMA 240: 443 (1978).
7. Kovick RB, Tillisch JH, Berens SC, Bramowitz AD, Shine KI: Vasodilator therapy of chronic left ventricular failure. Circulation 53: 322 (1976).
8. Packer M, Meller J, Gorlin R, Herman MV: Hemodynamic and clinical tachyphylaxis to prazosin-mediated afterload reduction in severe chronic congestive heart failure. Circulation 59: 531 (1979).
9. Steward DD: Remarkable tolerance to nitroglycerin. Philadelphia Polyclinic, 1888 August: 172.
10. Schelling J, Lasagna L: A study of cross-tolerance to circulatory effects of organic nitrates. Clin Pharmacol Ther 8: 256 (1967).
11. Zelis R, Mason DT: Isosorbide dinitrate. Effect on the vasodilator response to nitroglycerin. JAMA 234: 166 (1975).
12. Franciosa JA, Cohn JN: Sustained hemodynamic effects without tolerance during long-term isosorbide dinitrate treatment of chronic left ventricular failure. Am J Cardiol 45: 648 (1980).
13. Franciosa JA, Ragan DO, Rubenstone SJ: Validation of the CO_2 rebreathing method for measuring cardiac output in patients with hypertension or heart failure. J Lab Clin Med 88: 672 (1976).
14. Franciosa JA: Evaluation of the CO_2 rebreathing cardiac output method in seriously ill patients. Circulation 55: 449 (1977).

15. Rubin S, Chatterjee K, Gelbers HJ, Ports TA, Brundage BH, Parmley WW: Paradox of improved exercise but not resting hemodynamics with short-term prazosin in chronic heart failure. Am J Cardiol 43: 810 (1979).
16. Franciosa JA, Cohn JN: Effect of isosorbide dinitrate on response to submaximal and maximal exercise in patients with congestive heart failure. Am J Cardiol 43: 1009 (1979).
17. Franciosa JA, Goldsmith SR, Cohn JN: Contrasting immediate and long-term effects of isosorbide dinitrate on exercise capacity in congestive heart failure. Am J Med 69: 559 (1980).
18. Danahy DT, Burwell DT, Aronow WS, Prakash R: Sustained hemodynamic and antianginal effect of high dose oral isosorbide dinitrate. Circulation 55: 381 (1977).
19. Franciosa JA: Functional capacity of patients with chronic left ventricular failure: relationship of bicycle exercise performance to clinical and hemodynamic characterization. Am J Med 67: 460 (1979).
20. Franciosa JA, Park M, Levine TB: Lack of correlation between exercise capacity and indexes of resting left ventricular performance in heart failure. Am J Cardiol 47: 33 (1981).

Joseph A. Franciosa, M. D.
Cardiovascular Division – Slot 532
University of Arkansas for Medical Sciences
4301 West Markham Street
Little Rock, Arkansas 72205
U.S.A.

Discussion

BUSSMANN:

We did a similar study, but our results were not as positive as yours. We found less venodilatation in the chronic phase, despite some patients unproved clinically of the patients were markedly improved. In which way did your patients improve in their symptoms? Was there a change in classification?

FRANCIOSA:

For the group as a whole there was no significant change in clinical classification; the individuals did, but for the group there was no significant change.

Our feeling is that clinical classification is rather inadequate, as it is very subjective and we therefore prefer exercise testing for measuring responses. When we try to correlate clinical class using NYHA criteria with actually measured exercise performance, we find a very poor correlation between the two.

FOX:

In one patient the biggest fall of pulmonary wedge pressure occurred under placebo. Would you please comment on this?

FRANCIOSA:

I can only guess on that. First of all we have to do control studies. That particular patient had an alcoholic cardiomyopathy and my only guess is that we saw him in a very acute phase of his illness and he was spontaneously improving. We looked at him months later, his condition was much improved.

JÄHNCHEN:

Do you have any evidence that pharmacokinetics may be changed in patients with heart failure? Liver blood flow is reduced and this could cause a reduction in clearance.

FUNG:

We have done a study comparing the pharmacokinetics of oral isosorbide dinitrate in angina and congestive heart failure. There is no substantial change in the absorption and plasma concentrations.

ABRAMS:

At what time after medication did you measure the wedge pressure?

FRANCIOSA:

After 90 minutes.

ABRAMS:

Patients have been recatheterized or right-heart catheterizations were made after one to eight months of therapy. In every reported case a continued response has been found. One should measure the wedge pressure probably at 1, 2, 3, 4 and 5 hours.

FRANCIOSA:

I wish the wedge pressure had been measured in this study, unfortunately the arterial blood pressure was used. I am very sceptical about arterial pressure as an indicator of nitrate response. Our choice of timing is based largely on our previous experience with the first studies we did with isosorbide dinitrate. We just gave single doses and monitored hemodynamics, not pharmacokinetics, and found the peak effect about 90 minutes after oral dosing. The average duration of effect was of about 5 hours.

DEMARIA:

Presumably the major effect on the wedge pressure is the reduction in venous tone. Dr. Zelis's data regarding orthostatic changes would predominantly indicate that tolerance mainly concerned the venous bed.

FRANCIOSA:

Of course we are using the wedge pressure assuming that it is a reflection of venous dilation. But it may also reflect longterm changes in the afterload of the left ventricle which would also tend to reduce end-systolic volume and diastolic volume.
Data on pure arterial dilators clearly show no drop of the wedge pressure in long-term treatment. So I suspect that a minor part of the effect, not most of it, is on the venous side. This is contrary to Dr. Zelis's findings.

Hemodynamic Effects of 5-Isosorbide Mononitrate During Acute and Chronic Administration

M. Tauchert, W. Jansen, A. Osterspey, M. Fuchs, V. Hombach, H. H. Hilger

Introduction

Following the administration of isosorbide dinitrate (ISDN) to patients with coronary heart disease, pulmonary artery pressure, left-ventricular filling pressure, and myocardial oxygen consumption decline. As a result, patients experience a reduction in the frequency and severity of anginal attacks and their exercise tolerance increases. These acute effects of single doses of ISDN have been confirmed in numerous studies (2–4, 12, 13, 18, 23, 25–28).

The subsidance of ISDN-induced headaches, which are attributable to vasodilatation, during the course of long-term treatment led to the assumption of tolerance development soon after the introduction of ISDN therapy. The question has not yet been answered, however, whether tolerance during long-term ISDN treatment occurs uniformly and completely enough to jeopardize the value of chronic nitrate therapy (6, 8, 9, 12, 13, 17, 18, 21).

Two studies have been published regarding the development of tolerance during chronic administration of 5-isosorbide mononitrate (5-ISMN). We are aware only of the experimental study by Dietmann et al. (11) and the investigation by Smolarz et al. (24) in patients with coronary heart disease. Neither found evidence supporting the development of tolerance.

The objective of our investigation was to determine the hemodynamic effects of an acute initial dose of 5-ISMN in patients with coronary heart disease and to ascertain by means of follow-up measurements after a 4-week treatment period with 5-ISMN whether there was evidence of tolerance induced by chronic administration of the agent.

Patients and Methods

Investigated were 31 patients ranging in age from 42 to 62 years (mean 51.6 ± 5.6 years). Coronary heart disease had been verified in all patients by means of case history, exercise electrocardiogram, and coronary angiography. All antianginal drugs were discontinued prior to the study in accordance with their pharmacodynamic and pharmacokinetic properties. An exception was made in the case of chronic medication with cardiac glycosides. All investigative procedures were carried out during the early afternoon. The following hemodynamic parameters were determined at rest: heart rate; systolic, diastolic, and mean systemic blood pressure (Riva Rocci); and systolic, diastolic, and mean pulmonary artery pressure (right heart, flow-directed catheter). This was followed by supine bicycle ergometry at a workload of 50 W for 3 min. At the end of the 3rd exercise min, the aforementioned parameters were determined again. After a 15-min recovery period, during which heart rate, arterial blood pressure, and mean pulmonary artery pressure returned to their initial values, 12 patients (group I) received 20 mg 5-ISMN and the remaining 19 patients (group II) 50 mg 5-ISMN orally. All parameters were again measured 30 min after acute oral administration. This was followed by a second exercise test at the same workload as before mononitrate administration.

In ten patients from group II, the hemodynamic parameters measured at rest and during exercise for the initial workup were able to be redetermined after a 4-week monotherapy with 50 mg 5-ISMN three times daily. After the patients had taken their midday mononitrate dose (50 mg 5-ISMN), arterial blood pressure, pulmonary artery pressure, and heart rate were measured again. This was followed by an exercise test (50 W for 3 min) during which all parameters were again ascertained. Statistical analysis was carried out using Student's t-test for paired variables; significance was assumed at $p < 0.05$.

Results

The hemodynamic parameters before and after acute administration of 20 mg 5-ISDN are summarized in Table 1.

Hemodynamics Before and After 20 mg 5-ISMN

After acute administration of 20 mg 5-ISMN, systolic and diastolic arterial pressure at rest fell from 152 ± 15 to 140 ± 10 mmHg and 93 ± 11 to 90 ± 9 mmHg, respectively. No counterregulatory rise in heart rate was observed. Mean pulmonary artery pressure was reduced by about 25% (decline from 18.9 ± 5 to 14.2 ± 6 mmHg, $p < 0.001$).

The rise in systolic and diastolic blood pressure during exercise was significantly lower in the mononitrate than the control experiment (from 184 ± 8 to 178 ± 11 and 108 ± 14 to $\cdot102 \pm 11$ mmHg, respectively). Heart rate showed no consistent change. Mean pulmonary artery pressure fell markedly during exercise from 40.2 ± 9.1 to 30 ± 9 mmHg ($-25\%, p < 0.001$) (Fig. 1).

Hemodynamics Before and After 50 mg 5-ISMN

Systolic blood pressure fell significantly 30 min after the acute administration of 50 mg 5-ISMN (from 143 ± 19 to 131 ± 14 mmHg, $p < 0.01$); concomitantly, a reflex rise in heart rate was observed. Diastolic blood pressure remained unchanged. The 30% reduction in mean pulmonary artery pressure was considerably more pronounced than following the acute administration of 20 mg 5-ISMN (decline from 19.2 ± 6.6 to 13.5 ± 5.7 mmHg, $p < 0.001$). During exercise systolic, diastolic, and mean systemic arterial blood pressure declined significantly (from 172 ± 16 to 164 ± 19 mmHg systolic; 104 ± 12 to 97 ± 9 mmHg diastolic; 133 ± 13 to 126 ± 11 mmHg mean). Heart rate fell slightly (from 101 ± 15 to 97 ± 13 beats/min). Mean pulmonary artery pressure showed a reduction from 42.5 ± 14.8 to 25.3 ± 10.7 mmHg ($-40\%, p < 0.001$ (Fig. 2).

Table 1. Acute effect of 20 mg 5-isosorbide mononitrate (5-ISMN) on various hemodynamic parameters at rest and during exercise; mean values and SD in 12 patients with angiographically confirmed coronary heart disease

		Rest			Exercise		
		Control	5-ISMN acute	% difference	Control	5-ISMN acute	% difference
HR	(beats n/min)	73 ± 13	70 ± 18	−4% NS	102 ± 18	99 ± 17	−3% NS
RR_{syst}	(mmHg)	152 ± 15	140 ± 10	−8% *	184 ± 8	175 ± 11	−5% **
RR_{diast}	(mmHg)	93 ± 11	90 ± 9	−3% NS	108 ± 14	102 ± 11	−6% *
RR_{mean}	(mmHg)	119 ± 10	112 ± 8	−6% *	140 ± 8	134 ± 6	−4% NS
PAP_{syst}	(mmHg)	30 ± 5	21 ± 5	−31% ***	56 ± 13	44 ± 14	−21% **
PAP_{diast}	(mmHg)	13 ± 5	9 ± 5	−31% **	26 ± 8	22 ± 7	−15% *
PAP_{mean}	(mmHg)	18.9 ± 5	14.2 ± 6	−25% ***	40.2 ± 9.1	30 ± 9	−25% ***

* $p < 0.05$; ** $p < 0.01$; *** $p < 0.001$
HR, hear rate; RR_{syst}, systolic blood pressure; RR_{diast}, diastolic blood pressure; RR_{mean}, mean blood pressure; PAP_{syst}, systolic pulmonary artery pressure; PAP_{diast}, diastolic pulmonary artery pressure PAP_{mean}, mean pulmonary artery pressure

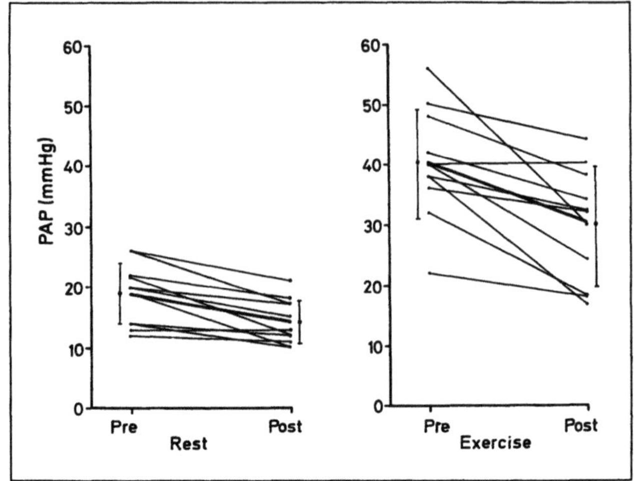

Fig. 1. Change in mean pulmonary artery pressure (*PAP*) following acute administration of 20 mg 5-isosorbide mononitrate at rest and during exercise (N = 12).

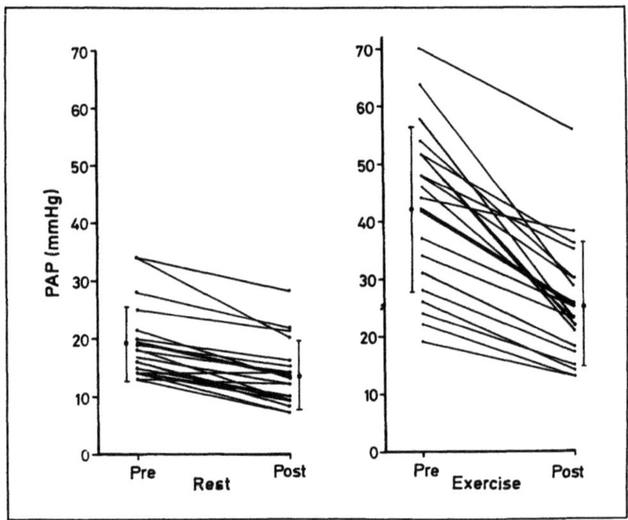

Fig. 2. Change in mean pulmonary artery pressure (*PAP*) following acute administration of 50 mg 5-isosorbide mononitrate at rest and during exercise (N = 19).

Long-Term Study: Hemodynamics Before and After 4-Week Maintenance Therapy with 50 mg 5-ISMN

The values obtained by hemodynamic measurements after chronic treatment with 50 mg 5-ISMN three times daily are summarized in Tables 3 and 4. Acute administration resulted in a reduction in both arterial and mean pulmonary artery blood pressure at rest and during exercise (at rest: systolic pressure, decline from 143 ± 21 to 128 ± 12 mmHg; mean pulmonary artery pressure, decline from 17 ± 3 to 12.2 ± 2.9 mmHg; during exercise: systolic blood pressure, decline from 173 ± 21 to 165 ± 21 mmHg; mean pulmonary artery pressure, decline from 42.4 ± 14 to 23.2 ± 6.8 mmHg); heart rate rose as a reflex response from 66 ± 9 to 72 ± 11 (Figs. 3 and 4).

46

Table 2. Acute effect of 20 mg 5-isosorbide mononitrate (5-ISMN) on various hemodynamic parameters at rest and during exercise; mean values and SD in 12 patients with angiographically confirmed coronary heart disease

		Rest			Exercise		
		Control	5-ISMN acute	% difference	Control	5-ISMN acute	% difference
HR	(beats n/min)	65 ± 9	72 ± 12	+10% **	101 ± 15	97 ± 13	−4% NS
RR_{syst}	(mmHg)	143 ± 19	131 ± 14	−8% **	172 ± 16	164 ± 19	−5% **
RR_{diast}	(mmHg)	90 ± 9	88 ± 8	−1% NS	104 ± 12	97 ± ± 9	−6% **
RR_{mean}	(mmHg)	112 ± 11	107 ± 9	−4% NS	133 ± 13	126 ± 11	−5% *
PAP_{syst}	(mmHg)	30 ± 8	20 ± 6	−31% ***	57 ± 19	38 ± 13	−33% ***
PAP_{diast}	(mmHg)	12.5 ± 5	10.2 ± 4.8	−17% **	24.8 ± 10	16.7 ± 9	−33% ***
PAP_{mean}	(mmHg)	19.2 ± 6.6	13.5 ± 5.7	−30% ***	42.5 ± 14.8	25.3 ± 10.7	−40% ***

* $p < 0.05$; ** $p < 0.01$; *** $p < 0.001$

HR, hear rate; RR_{syst}, systolic blood pressure; RR_{diast}, diastolic blood pressure; RR_{mean}, mean blood pressure; PAP_{syst}, systolic pulmonary artery pressure; PAP_{diast}, diastolic pulmonary artery pressure PAP_{mean}, mean pulmonary artery pressure

Table 3. Effects of acute and chronic treatment with 5-ISMN (50 mg three times a day) on various hemodynamic parameters at rest and during exercise; mean values and SD in ten patients with angiographically confirmed coronary heart disease

		Rest			Exercise		
		Control	5-ISMN acute	5-ISMN chronic	Control	5-ISMN acute	5-ISMN chronic
Hr	(beats n/min)	66 ± 9	72 ± 11	68 ± 10	107 ± 17	99 ± 11	104 ± 14
RR_{syst}	(mmHg)	143 ± 21	128 ± 12	134 ± 15	173 ± 21	165 ± 21	176 ± 17
RR_{diast}	(mmHg)	91 ± 9	88 ± 7	86 ± 11	105 ± 12	97 ± 9	102 ± 12
RR_{mean}	(mmHg)	113 ± 13	105 ± 8	107 ± 12	134 ± 15	126 ± 13	133 ± 15
PAP_{syst}	(mmHg)	26 ± 5	20 ± 6	21 ± 6	60 ± 19	36 ± 9	48 ± 18
PAP_{diast}	(mmHg)	11 ± 3.7	9.2 ± 2.5	8.5 ± 2.8	27.9 ± 8.3	16.4 ± 7	23.5 ± 11.1
AP_{mean}	(mmHg)	17 ± 3	12.2 ± 2.9	12.7 ± 3.6	42.2 ± 14	23.2 ± 6.8	36.2 ± 16.3

* $p < 0.05$; ** $p < 0.01$; *** $p < 0.001$

HR, heart rate; RR_{syst}, systolic blood pressure; RR_{diast}, diastolic blood pressure; RR_{mean}, mean blood pressure; PAP_{syst}, systolic pulmonary artery pressure; PAP_{diast}, diastolic pulmonary artery pressure; PAP_{mean}, mean pulmonary artery pressure

Table 4. Effects of acute and chronic treatment with 5-ISMN (50 mg three times a day) in various hemodynamic parameters at rest and during exercise; percentage change and statistical significance

	Rest			Exercise		
	Control/ acute	Control/ chronic	Acute/ chronic	Control/ acute	Control/ chronic	Acute/ chronic
HR	+9% NS	+3% NS	−5.6% NS	−7.5% *	−3% NS	+5% NS
RR_{syst}	−10% *	−6% NS	+4.7% NS	−4.6% NS	+2% NS	+7% NS
RR_{diast}	−3% NS	−5% NS	−2% NS	−7.6% **	−3% NS	+5% NS
RR_{mean}	−7% *	−5% NS	+2% NS	−6% **	−1% NS	+6% NS
PAP_{syst}	−23% ***	−19% **	+5% NS	−40% ***	−20% **	+33% *
PAP_{diast}	−16% **	−23% *	−7% *	−41% ***	−16% NS	+43% NS
PAP_{mean}	−28% ***	−25% **	+4% NS	−45% ***	−14% *	+56% *

HR, heart rate; RR_{syst}, systolic blood pressure; RR_{diast}, diastolic blood pressure; RR_{mean}, mean blood pressure; PAP_{syst}, systolic pulmonary artery pressure; PAP_{diast}, diastolic pulmonary artery pressure; PAP_{mean}, mean pulmonary artery pressure

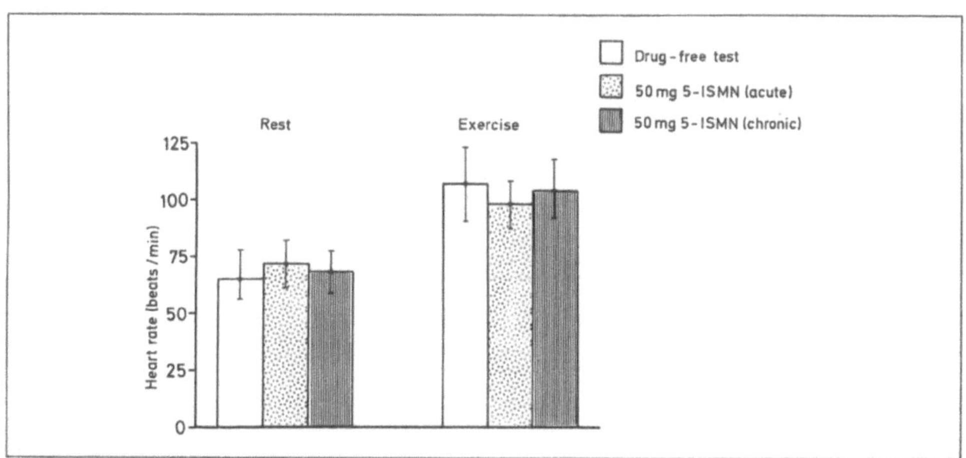

Fig. 3. Change in heart rate during acute and long-term treatment with 5-isosorbide mononitrate (*5-ISMN*) at rest and during exerise (N = 10).

After 4 weeks of long-term treatment with 50 mg 5-ISMN three times daily the renewed acute administration of 50 mg 5-ISMN resulted in a slight, insignificant decline in blood pressure and rise in heart rate compared to control values (reduction in systolic blood pressure to 134 ± 15 mmHg at rest, rise in heart rate to 68 ± 10 beats/min). Mean pulmonary artery pressure at rest showed an approximately 20% decline following mononitrate administration (fall from 15.8 ± 3 to 12.7 ± 2.9 mmHg, $p < 0.001$). During ergometry, no change in heart rate and blood pressure was observed in comparison to control values obtained prior to long-term therapy (Figs. 3 and 4). Mean pulmonary artery pressure reduction during exercise was only 14%. During exercise with long-term medication, the decline in mean pulmonary artery pressure was markedly less pronounced than in the acute experiment (acute administration, 40%, chronic therapy, 14%) (Fig. 5).

49

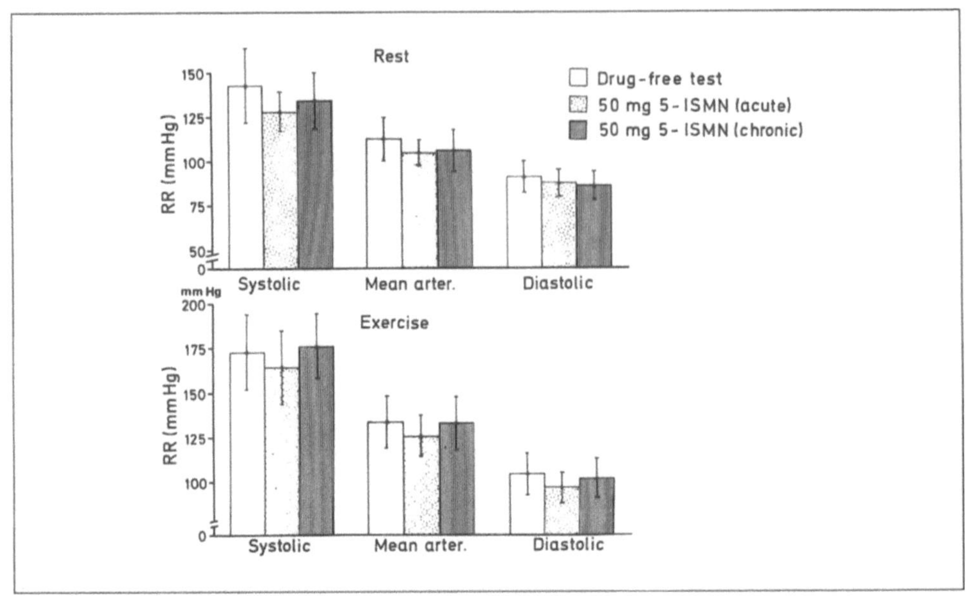

Fig. 4. Change in systolic, diastolic, and mean arterial blood pressure (*RR*) during acute and long-term treatment with 5-isosorbide mononitrate (*5-ISMN*) at rest and during exercise.

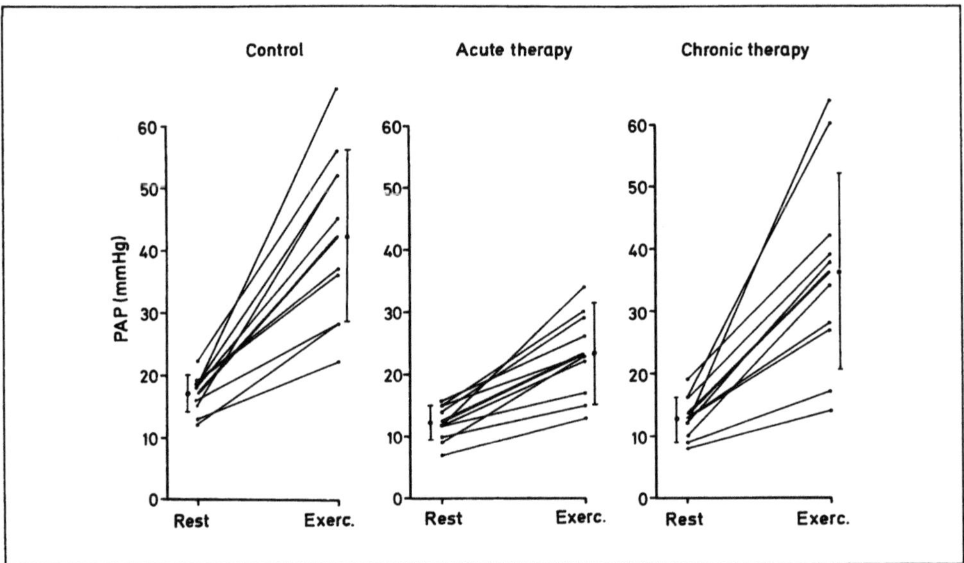

Fig. 5. Change in mean pulmonary artery pressure (*PAP*) during acute and long-term treatment with 50 mg 5-isosorbide mononitrate (*5-ISMN*) at rest and during exercise (*Exerc.*). (10 patients out of group II, before and after chronic treatment with 50 mg 5-ISMN three times daily.)

Discussion

When adequate dosages are used, there are no significant differences between ISDN and its metabolites in terms of antianginal efficacy (7, 23, 26). Both mononitrates display considerably longer half-lives than ISDN (1, 11, 23, 26). Determinations of 5-ISMN plasma levels demonstrate that its effective concentration is subject to slighter variations than the effective levels of ISDN and its metabolites (1). Variations in resorption of between 44% and 76% of the administered dose have been observed following oral ISDN therapy, whereas interindividual variations after 5-ISMN are five times lower (1).

In light of these pharmacokinetic differences, it seems appropriate to replace ISDN with 5-ISMN in long-term nitrate therapy. Our findings confirm the already known hemodynamic effects of 5-ISMN (5, 7, 14, 19, 23–26). As with ISDN (4, 27, 28) or nitroglycerin (15, 16), systolic and diastolic blood pressure at rest and during exercise fell slightly following acute oral administration of 5-ISMN. Resting heart rate rose significantly after only 50 mg 5-ISMN. Compared to the effect of a 20-mg dose of 5-ISMN, the decline in mean pulmonary artery pressure following 50 mg 5-ISMN was considerably more pronounced (at rest: −25% vs −30%; during exercise −25% vs −40%).

There have been no studies concerning the possible development of tolerance after long-term therapy, such as have been carried out for nitroglycerin and ISDN with controversial results (3, 6, 8–10, 12, 13, 17, 18, 20–22, 29), with the exception of the work of Dietmann et al. (11) and Smolarz et al. (24). Smolarz et al., using the parameters heart rate, blood pressure, and double product, found no evidence of tolerance development after a 2-month treatment period with 20 mg 5-ISMN twice or three times a day.

In our ten patients with coronary heart disease who received long-term treatment, an acute dose of 50 mg 5-ISMN resulted in a slight reduction in arterial blood pressure and a marked decline in mean pulmonary artery pressure at rest (18.9 ± 5 to 14.2 ± 6 mmHg, $p < 0.001$). After 4 weeks of uninterrupted therapy, heart rate and arterial blood pressure did not change significantly in response to an acute single dose of 50 mg 5-ISMN prior to the follow-up experiments. Mean pulmonary artery pressure at rest was lower during maintenance therapy than prior to the onset of treatment; the renewed acute administration of 50 mg 5-ISMN yielded a further reduction in pressure of 20% (vs 28% before long-term therapy). This suggests that the effect on venous pooling was attenuated but still clearly demonstrable. Under exercise conditions, the therapeutic effect of nitrates is even more evident: the acute administration of 50 mg 5-ISMN led to a 45% decline in pulmonary artery pressure compared to values obtained without medication. This effect was significantly attenuated following chronic treatment with 50 mg 5-ISMN three times a day (pulmonary artery pressure reduction of only 14% compared to untreated controls) (Fig. 6). Heart rate and arterial blood pressure were no longer affected by acute administration of the agent during long-term therapy. Thus conscientiously administered high-dose maintenance therapy with 5-ISMN apparently results in significant tolerance development. The concept of various authors that the development of nitrate tolerance applies only to the arterial system (12, 13, 18) must be questioned on the basis of our findings.

Principally biochemical mechanisms have been discussed as causes of the development of tolerance to vasodilators. Needleman and Johnson (29) attribute it to the oxidation of sulfur hydroxide-bearing receptors in the vicinity of regulatory vessels. Lichtlen (18) postulates stimulation of the renin-angiotension-aldosterone system with resultant counterregulation in the venous system.

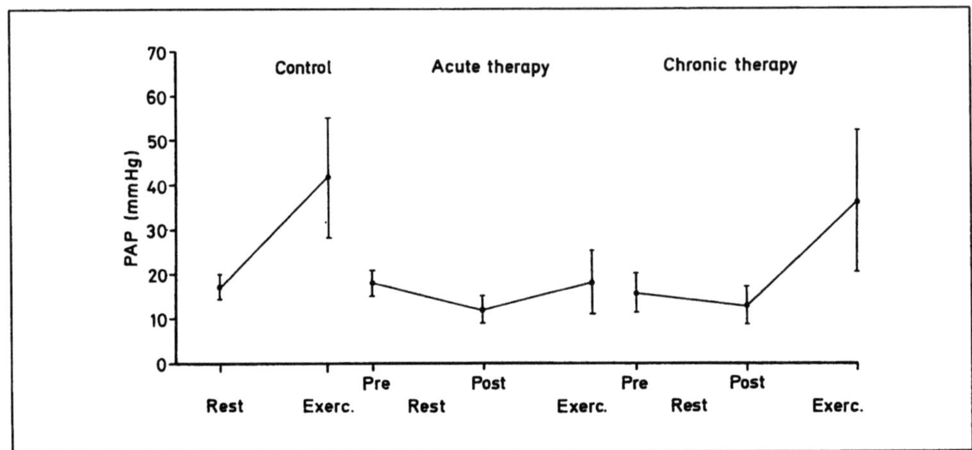

Fig. 6. Mean pulmonary artery pressure (*PAP*) at rest and during exercise (*Exerc.*) (ergometry: 50 W for 3 min). *Left,* before medication; *center,* value at rest–value at rest following 50 mg 5-ISMN–ergometry following 50 mg 5-ISMN; *right,* value at rest during chronic therapy–value at rest following 50 mg 5-ISMN during chronic therapy–ergometry following 50 mg 5-ISMN during chronic therapy.

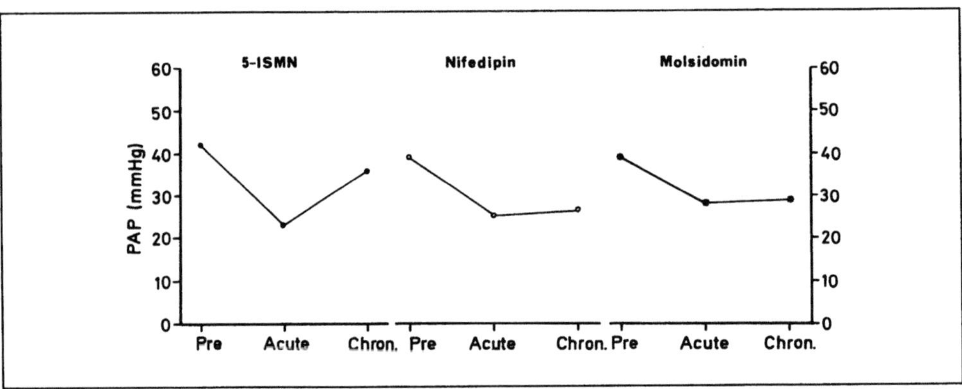

Fig. 7. Change in mean pulmonary artery pressure (*PAP*) during exercise (*Exerc.*) (ergometry 50 W for 3 min) during long-term therapy with a 50 mg 5-isosorbide mononitrate (*5-ISMN*) three times a day. 20 mg nifedipine three times a day, and 2 mg molsidomine three times a day.

Our own ongoing studies fail to indicate the development of comparable tolerance during chronic therapy with nifedipine and molsidomine (Fig. 7). This observation comes unexpectedly with regard to molsidomine, since the drug's mechanisms of action are thought to be similar to those of the nitrates (28).

The intentionally high dosage of 5-ISMN that we employed suggests that the optimum dosage of the agent was exceeded. Our findings, however, cast doubt upon whether the recently pursued objective of attaining the highest and most constant plasma nitrate levels possible is really meaningful in the development of such pharmaceuticals.

References

1. Abshagen U, Spörl-Radun S, Betzien G, Kaufmann B, Endele R: Pharmakokinetik, Wirkung und Verträglichkeit von Isosorbiddinitrat, Isosorbid-5-Mononitrat bei gesunden Versuchspersonen. Med. Welt 32: 509 (1981).
2. Aronow WS, Chesluk HM: Evaluation of nitroglycerin in angina in patients on isosorbide dinitrate. Circulation 42: 61 (1970).
3. Becker HJ, Walden G, Kaltenbach M: Gibt es eine Tachyphylaxie beziehungsweise Gewöhnung bei der Behandlung der Angina pectoris mit Nitrokörpern? Verh Dtsch Ges Inn Med 82: 1208 (1976).
4. Behrenbeck DW, Tauchert M, Niehues B, Hilger HH: Der Einfluß einer „afterload-Verminderung" auf den Sauerstoffverbrauch des Myokards. Verh Dtsch Ges Kreislaufforschg 42: 286 (1976).
5. Biamino G, Oeff M, Andresen D, Lichey HJ, Prokein E, Arntz R, Leitner E, Schröder R: Hämodynamische Effekte von Isosorbid-5-mononitrat unter Ruhe- und Belastungsbedingungen bei Patienten mit schwerer Angina pectoris. Med Welt 32: 535 (1981).
6. Blasini R, Brügmann U, Mannes A, Froer KL, Hall D, Rudolph W: Wirksamkeit von Isosorbiddinitrat in retardierter Form bei Langzeitbehandlung. Herz 5: 298 (1980).
7. Bödigheimer K, Nowak FG, Delius W: Vergleichende invasive Untersuchung über die Wirkung von Isosorbid-5-Mononitrat und Isosorbiddinitrat bei chronischer Herzinsuffizienz. Med Welt 32: 543 (1981).
8. Bubenheimer P, Hauf GF, Haas J, Roskamm H: Behandlung der Stauungsherzinsuffizienz mit Vasodilatatoren. Abhängigkeit der hämodynamischen Effekte von einer vorausgegangenen Vasodilatatoren-Medikation. Z Kardiol 69: 202 (1980).
9. Danahy DT, Aronow WS: Hemodynamic and antianginal effect of high dose oral isosorbide dinitrate after chronic use. Circulation 56: 205 (1977).
10. Davidov ME, Mcroczek WJ: Effect of sustained release nitroglycerin capsules on anginal frequency and exercise capacity. A double-blind-evaluation. Angiology 28: 181 (1977).
11. Dietmann K, Sponer G, Voss E: Pharmakodynamik, Pharmakokinetik und Metabolismus der Nitrate des Isosorbids am wachen Hund. Med Welt 32: 481 (1981).
12. Franciosa JA, Cohn JY: Sustained hemodynamic effect without tolerance during long-term Isosorbide dinitrate treatment of chronic left ventricular failure. Am J Cardiol 45: 648 (1980).
13. Hauf GF, Bubenheimer P, Lönne E, Roskamm H: Behandlung der Stauungsherzinsuffizienz mit Vasodilatatoren. Vergleich der Akut- und Langzeiteffekte unter Berücksichtigung verschiedener Substanzgruppen. Dtsch Med Wschr 106: 1607 (1981).
14. Isbary J, Doering W, Wauer B, Greding H, König E: Hämodynamische Veränderungen in Ruhe und während Belastung nach 20 mg Isosorbid-5-Mononitrat bei Patienten mit koronarer Herzkrankheit, Med Welt 32: 531 (1981).
15. Jansen W, Niehues B, Tauchert M, Hombach V, Behrenbeck DW, Hilger HH: Die Änderung der Koronardurchblutung und des myokardialen Sauerstoffverbrauches in Ruhe und bei Belastung nach Gabe von Nitroglycerin im Vergleich zu Tenormin, einem kardioselektiven Beta-Rezeptorenblocker. Verh Dtsch Ges Inn Med 86: 593 (1980).
16. Jansen W, Hombach V, Tauchert M, Niehues B, Behrenbeck DW, Hilger HH: Der Einfluß von Nitroglycerin auf die Koronardurchblutung und den myokardialen Sauerstoffverbrauch bei körperlicher Belastung. Herz/Kreislauf 13: 313 (1981).
17. Lee G, Mason DT, DeMaria AN: Effects of long-term oral administration of isosorbide dinitrate on the antianginal response to nitroglycerin. Absence of nitrate cross tolerance and self tolerance shown by exercise testing. Am J Cardiol 41: 82 (1978).
18. Lichtlen PR: Langzeitnitrate bei Angina Pectoris. Gibt es eine Toleranz-Entwicklung? Münch Med Wschr 122: 1753 (1980).
19. Mehmel HC, Ruffmann K, Schwarz F, Manthey J, Kübler W: Die Wirkung von Isosorbid-5-Mononitrat (IS-5-MN) auf die linksventrikuläre Hämodynamik. Med Welt 32: 527 (1981).
20. Needleman P, Johnson EM: Mechanism of tolerance development to organic nitrates. J Pharmacol Exp Ther 184: 709 (1973).
21. Parker JO, Thadani U: Tolerance to circulatory and clinical effects of nitrates. In: Nitrates III. Cardiovascular Effects. Ed. PR Lichtlen, Engel HJ, Schrey A, Swan HJC. Springer-Verlag (Berlin–Heidelberg–New York) (1981), S 27.

22. Schelling J, Lasagna L: A study to cross tolerance to circulatory effects of organic nitrates. Clin Pharmacol Ther 8: 256 (1967).
23. Seidel F, Michel D: Comparative hemodynamic and pharmacokinetic investigation after oral isosorbide-2-mononitrate and isosorbide-5-mononitrate. In: Nitrates III, Cardiovascular Effects, Ed. P R Lichtlen Engel HJ, Schrey A, Swan HJC. Springer-Verlag (Berlin–Heidelberg–New York) (1981), S. 54.
24. Smorlarz A, Seeliger S, Glocker M: Langzeitverträglichkeit und Wirkung von Isosorbid-5-Mononitrat (IS-5-MN) bei Patienten mit koronarer Herzkrankheit. Med Welt 32: 549 (1981).
25. Stauch M, Grewe N, Nissen H: Die Wirkung von 2- und 5-Isosorbidmononitrat auf das Belastungs-EKG bei Patienten mit Koronarinsuffizienz. Verh Dtsch Ges Kreislaufforschg 41: 181 (1975).
26. Stauch M, Grewe N: Die Wirkung von Isosorbiddinitrat, Isosorbid-2- und 5-Mononitrat auf das Belastungs-EKG und die Hämodynamik während Vorhofstimulation bei Patienten mit Angina pectoris. Z Kardiol 68: 687 (1979).
27. Tauchert M, Behrenbeck DW, Hilger HH: Der Einfluß von Nitraten auf Hämodynamik und myokardialen Sauerstoffverbrauch. In: Schettler G, Horsch A, Mörl H, Orth H, Weizel A: Der Herzinfarkt, Schattauer-Verlag (Stuttgart-New York), S. 332.
28. Tauchert M, Behrenbeck DW, Niehues B, Jansen W, Carstens V, Hilger HH: Nitroglycerin und Isosorbiddinitrat als Referenzsubstanzen bei der Prüfung koronarwirksamer Pharmaka. In: Rudolph W, Schrey A (Hrsg), Nitrate II, Wirkung auf Herz und Kreislauf, Urban & Schwarzenberg (München–Wien–Baltimore) (1980) S. 82.
29. Thadani U, Manyari D, Parker JO, Fung HL: Tolerance to the circulatory effects of oral isosorbide dinitrate. Rate of development and cross-tolerance to glyceryl trinitrate. Circulation 61: 526 (1980).

Authors' address:
Prof. Dr. M. Tauchert
Medizinische Universitäts-Klinik
und Poliklinik
Innere Medizin III – Kardiologie
Joseph-Stelzmann-Str. 9
5000 Köln 41

Discussion

FRANCIOSA:

I have to bring up again the same question of sympathetic stimulation. Your range of pulmonary pressures was quite wide. In some of your patients the mean pulmonary artery pressure went down to 10 or 12, some to 20 or 30 mm Hg. I think we would all agree that in patients with low filling pressure or with low wedge pressure nitrates can produce a very marked drop in stroke volume with consecutive very marked tachycardia and other sympathetic responses.
I wonder if you have investigated separately the response in those patients whose pulmonary pressures were quite low, to look for changes in the long run in terms of heart rate, blood pressure, body weight and so forth.

TAUCHERT:

The question of sympathetic activation was not tested. I think it is important these patients only received 5-nitrate. They could use nitroglycerin in anginal attacks, but nothing else. There were no significant changes in heart rate, blood pressure or body weight.

DEMARIA:

May I ask you to comment on the differences of your results compared with those of Dr. Franciosa?

TAUCHERT:

One reason could be the fact that no other drugs were given. In a former study we saw acute reactivation of the nitroglycerin response by furosemide. We did not use diuretics while your patients received such products. Another point is the longer duration of action of high doses of 5-nitrate. So its effects lasted for about 24 h with no possibility of recovery of any mechanism. A further point was that we made the first measurement after initiating the treatment.

KALTENBACH:

How far did the increase in mean pulmonary arterial pressure indicate myocardial ischemia? Was this a point at which the patients experienced angina, and did you use individualized work loads, or was it just a work load of 50 watt for all patients, regardless of whether they had angina, so that the increase in pulmonary arterial pressure could also be indicative of some ventricular dysfunction and not necessarily of myocardial ischemia?

TAUCHERT:

The maximal work load during chronic doses was nearly the same as at control. In the acute experiment the maximal work load attained was higher with nitrates, but not after long-term treatment. The patients' complaints were the same with and without medication. We used a standard load of 50 watt for three minutes, but afterwards we increased to maximal load.

ABRAMS:

Many pharmaceutical companies have tried to increase the duration of nitrate action by sustained release forms or by increasing the single dose. If in fact Dr. Tauchert's hypothesis is correct, we should
not go on with our efforts to have a strong nitrate effect around the clock.

Investigations to Demonstrate Nitrate Tolerance in Peripheral Vessels by Means of a Simple Hemodynamic Test

P. Schlup, C. Zatti, H. Studer

Introduction

The possibility of tolerance development during nitrate therapy is raised repeatedly in the literature (1–6). We asked ourselves whether a loss of efficacy during long-term nitrate therapy could be identified by means of a simple hemodynamic test possibly even suitable for use on an outpatient basis. We also attempted to answer the question of whether an eventual loss of drug efficacy was due to true tolerance development or was merely an apparent phenomenon in the context of adaptive changes.

The primary effect of the nitrates is to relax smooth muscles in peripheral vessels (5, 7). The resulting vasodilatation can be identified using simple clinical investigations, such as measurements of the decline in systolic blood pressure and rise in heart rate, and finger plethysmography (8–10). The quotient of maximal systolic and minimal diastolic flow can be calculated oscillometrically (Fig. 1). The greater the quotient, the more pronounced the vasodilatation. In addition, the difference is more marked in the standing position than in the sitting position (11).

Subjects and Methods

We determined heart rate and blood pressure and carried out finger plethysmography in eight young, healthy probands (mean age 28 years) at intervals of 1–5 min. Measurements were taken in the supine and standing positions immediately before and after the sublingual administration of 1.6 mg nitroglycerin. The first test was performed before and a second test after a 3-day course of 20 mg isosorbide dinitrate (ISDN) three times daily. In a second series of tests we investigated ten patients with angina pectoris (mean age 62 years) at the onset of treatment with 60–100 mg ISDN per day and again after an average of 12 weeks.

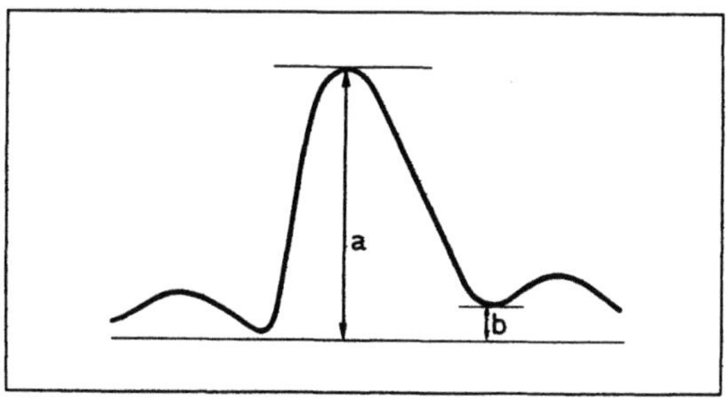

Fig. 1. Quotient of maximal systolic (*a*) and minimal diastolic (*b*) flow: a/b.

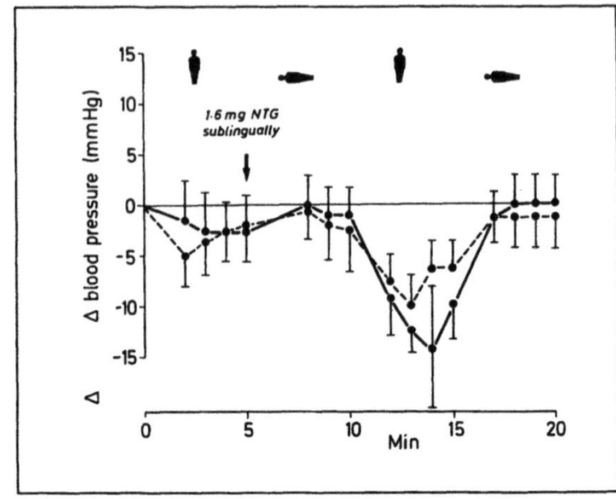

Fig. 2. Blood pressure in healthy subjects (N = 8). *Solid line,* before, and *broken line,* after isosorbide dinitrate; *NTG,* nitroglycerin.

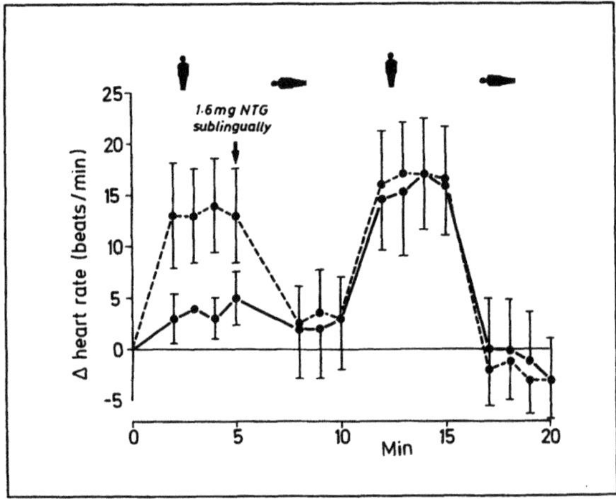

Fig. 3. Heart rate in healthy subjects (N = 8). *Solid line,* before, and *broken line,* after isosorbide dinitrate; *NTG,* nitroglycerin.

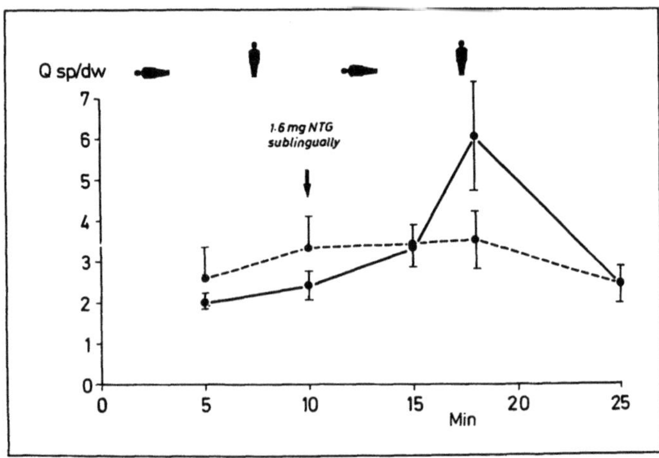

Fig. 4. Plethysmography (acral oscillogram) in healthy subjects (N = 8). *Solid line,* before, and *broken line,* after isosorbide dinitrate; *NTG,* nitroglycerin.

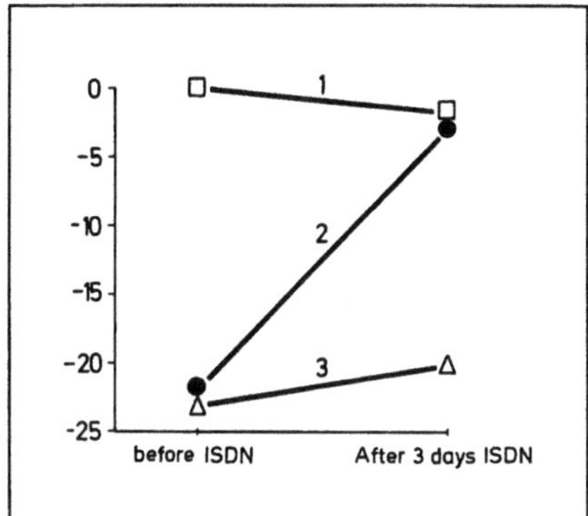

Fig. 5. Individual response to nitrates in three healthy subjects: systolic blood pressure during orthostasis after 1.6 mg nitroglycerin sublingually. *ISDN*, isosorbide dinitrate.

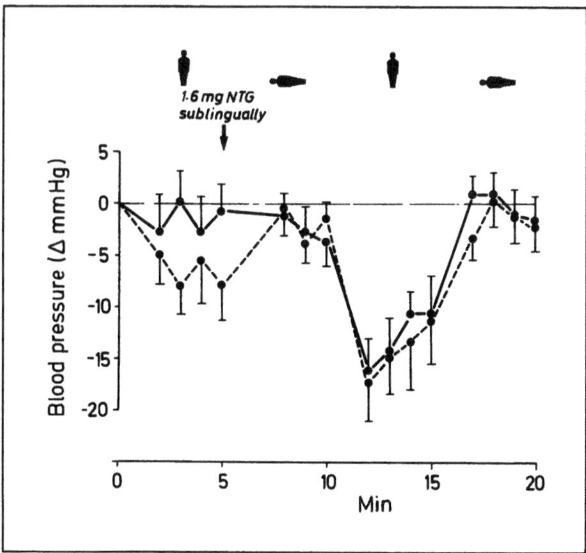

Fig. 6. Blood pressure in patients with angina pectoris (N = 10). *Solid line*, patients receiving isosorbide dinitrate (*ISDN*) during first test; *broken line*, patients receiving ISDN during second test; *NTG*, nitroglycerin.

Results
Healthy Probands

The orthostatic decline in blood pressure was much more pronounced following nitroglycerin. A 3-day pretreatment phase with ISDN did not affect the blood pressure response (Fig. 2). Following nitroglycerin heart rate rose much higher in response to orthostasis than previously. A 3-day pretreatment phase resulted in the same orthostatic heart rate increase as in the previous acute test. The difference was significant. With renewed administration of nitroglycerin, therefore, no increase in heart rate was discernible (Fig. 3). The plethysmographically determined quotient rose significantly in both the supine and standing positions following nitroglycerin. No further vasodilatation was seen in an acute test after a 3-day treatment with ISDN (Fig. 4). The great interindividual variability of the nitrate effect (Fig. 5) was noticeable.

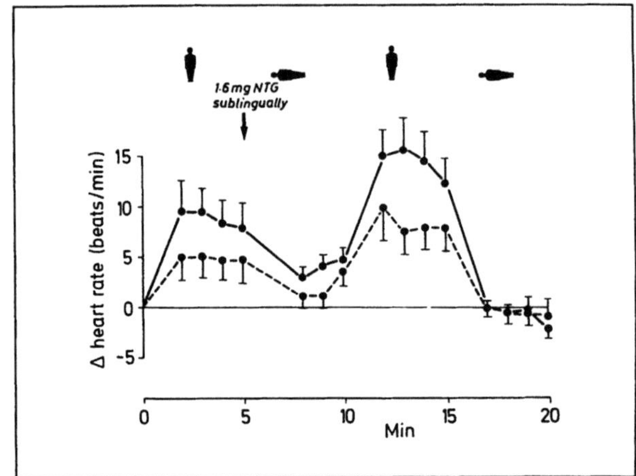

Fig. 7. Heart rate in patients with angina pectoris (N = 10). *Solid line,* patients receiving isosorbide dinitrate (*ISDN*) during first test; *broken line,* patients receiving ISDN during second test; *NTG,* nitroglycerin.

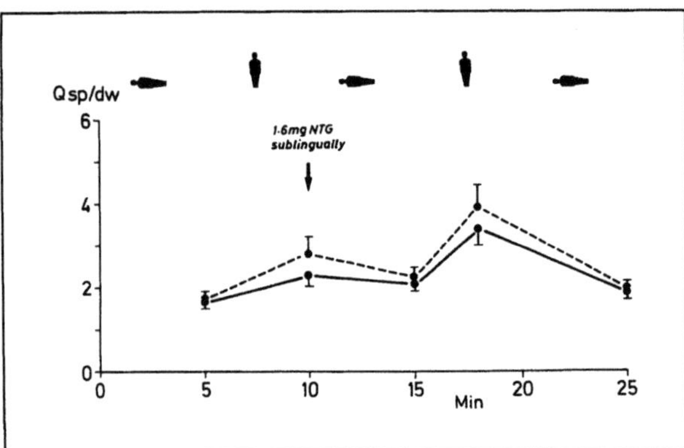

Fig. 8. Plethysmography (acral oscillogram) in patients with angina pectoris (N = 10). *Solid line,* patients receiving isosorbide dinitrate (*ISDN*) during first test; *broken line,* patients receiving *ISDN* during second test; *NTG,* nitroglycerin.

Patients with Angina Pectoris

In the standing position, the blood pressure response in the patients was virtually identical to that in the healthy subjects. The marked orthostatic decline in blood pressure following nitroglycerin was not significantly attenuated even after a 3-month course of ISDN (Fig. 6). The orthostatic increase in heart rate declined progressively as the duration of therapy increased; the difference in heart rate while standing became significant (Fig. 7). The patients also responded to the additional administration of nitroglycerin with oscillometrically verifiable vasodilatation. In contrast to the case in the healthy subjects, the extent of this response remained virtually unchanged after 12 weeks of treatment (Fig. 8).

Discussion

Numerous experimental studies in animals have shown that repeated exposure to organic nitrates results in a reduction in their pharmacological effect on peripheral vessels

60

(12–17, 36). The results of investigations in man are more contradictory (18–23). Clinically relevant tolerance to the favorable effects of nitrates on angina pectoris (4, 18, 24–27) and severe congestive heart failure (28–25) has not yet been documented. Our findings speak against the development of tolerance in peripheral vessels. On the basis of differing results in short- and long-term tests, the following hypothesis can be formulated. After brief, uninterrupted nitrate treatment compensatory processes still remain extremely pronounced, since the sympathetic nervous system is maximally stimulated by the nitrate-induced vasodilatation. For the physiologically most important parameter – namely systemic blood pressure – to remain stable, heart rate must be increased and the peripheral vascular system again constricted. Our findings in the healthy subjects point in this direction. Following a 3-day treatment period with ISDN, orthostasis alone, even before the additional nitrate administration, caused a significantly greater increase in heart rate. Actually, the orthostatic fall in blood pressure was no greater than prior to the onset of treatment. If, however, the pharmacological effect of ISDN was potentiated by the acute administration of nitroglycerin in the same subjects, a blood pressure decline to dangerous levels during orthostasis could only be prevented if vasoconstriction occurred. This might explain why in this setting additional vasodilatation was absent oscillometrically. If the therapy lasts some time, the circulation adapts. A new equilibrium is established. Blood pressure remains unchanged, although the orthostatic increase in heart rate is reduced. In addition, the extent of reflex vasoconstriction during orthostasis following acute nitroglycerin administration declined. The degree of vasodilation remained virtually unchanged oscillometrically after 12 weeks.

It is obvious that the results and our conclusions might have been different with a greater number of patients, a larger dose of ISDN, and a longer treatment period. The wide variation in the measured values is indicative of this. To a great extent it is attributable to the marked interindividual variability in the effect of nitrate administration. This interesting phenomenon has been observed only rarely to date.

Summary

Following a 3-day course of ISDN in healthy subjects no attenuation of the effect of nitroglycerin on heart rate and blood pressure occurred. By contrast, a significant decline in nitrate-induced vasodilatation was measurable plethysmographically. When patients with coronary heart disease were treated for 3 months with ISDN, the results were somewhat different. In an acute test with nitroglycerin, the orthostatic increase in heart rate was significantly reduced. The response of blood pressure, however, did not change and was virtually identical to the degree of vasodilatation after 12 weeks. We therefore found no hard evidence supporting the development of tolerance in peripheral vessels.

References

1. Becker HJ et al: Gibt es eine „Tachyphylaxie" beziehungsweise Gewöhnung bei der Behandlung der Angina pectoris mit Nitrokörpern? Verh dtsch Ges inn Med 82: 1208 (1976).
2. Cohen S: The volatile Nitrites. JAMA 241: 2077 (1979).
3. Danahy DT et al: Sustained hemodynamic and antianginal effect of high dose oral Isosorbide Dinitrate. Circulation 55: 381 (1977).

4. Goldstein RE and Epstein S: Nitrates in the prophylactic treatment of Angina pectoris. Circulation 48: 917 (1973).
5. Kaltenbach M und Becker HJ: Nitrate in der Therapie der koronaren Herzkrankheit. DMW 104: 1723 (1979).
6. Nickerson M: Vasodilator drugs. In: The pharmacological basis of therapeutics (Goodman LS and Giman A (Ed)) 5, 727. MacMillan Publishing Co. Inc. New York 1975.
7. Becker K, Pitt B: Regional blood flow, ischemia and antianginal drugs. Ann Clin Res 3, 353 (1971).
8. Bollinger A et al: Die Wirkung von Isosorbiddinitrat auf den peripheren Kreislauf: eine Studie mit kontinuierlicher perkutaner Flußmessung in der A. femoralis. In: Nitrate I (Rudolf W., Siegenthaler W (Ed)) 54–60. Urban und Schwarzenberg, München–Berlin–Wien 1976.
9. Klepzig H: Veränderungen der Hämodynamik in der Peripherie unter der Einwirkung von Nitrokörpern. In: Nitrate I, Rudolf W, Siegenthaler W, (Ed)) 62: Urban und Schwarzenberg München–Berlin–Wien 1976.
10. Morikawa Y et al: Organic Nitrates poisoning at an explosives factory. Plethysmographic study. Arch Environ Health 14: 614 (1967.
11. Wei JY et al.: Relation of time course of plasma nitroglycerin levels to echocardiographic, arterial pressure and heart rate changes after sublingual administration of nitroglycerin. Amer J Cardiol 48, 778 (1981).
12. Crandall CA et al: The fate of glyceryltrinitrate in the tolerant and nontolerant animal. J Pharmacol Exp Ther 48: 127 (1933).
13. Herman AG and Bogaert MG: Organic nitrates: tolerance at the level of the vascular smooth muscle. Arch int Pharmacodyn 192: 200 (1971).
14. Myers H and Austin V Thomas: Nitrite toleration. J Pharmacol and Exper Ther 36: 227 (1929).
15. Needleman P: Tolerance to the vascular effects of Glyceryl-trinitrate. J Pharmacol and Exper Ther 171: 98 (1970).
16. Needleman P and Johnson E: Mechanism of tolerance development to organic nitrates. J Pharmacol and Exper Ther 184: 709 (1973).
17. Needleman P and Johnson E: The pharmacological and biochemical interaction of organic nitrates with sulfhydrils: possible correlations with the mechanism of tolerance development, vasodilation, and mitrochondrial and enzyme reactions. In: Handbook of experimental Pharmacology (Needleman P (Ed)) 97–104. Springer Verlag New York Inc. 1975.
18. Danahy DT and Aronow WS: Hemodynamic and antianginal effects of high dose oral Isosorbide Dinitrate after chronic use. Circulation 56: 206 (1977).
19. Goldstein RE et al: Clinical and circulatory effects of Isosorbide Dinitrate. Comparison with Nitroglycerin. Circulation 43: 629 (1971).
20. Schelling JC and Lasagna L: A study of cross tolerance to circulatory effects of organic nitrates. Clin Pharmacol Ther 8: 256 (1966).
21. Thadani U et al: Tolerance to the circulatory effects of oral Isosorbide-Dinitrate. Circulation 61: 526 (1980).
22. Zelis R and Mason DT: Demonstration of Nitrite tolerance: attenuation of the venodilator response to nitroglycerin to the chronic administration of Isosorbide Dinitrate. Circulation, Suppl III to 39 and 40, 221 (1969).
23. Zelis R and Mason DT: Isosorbide Dinitrate Effect on the vasodilator response to nitroglycerin. JAMA 234: 166 (1975).
24. Aronow WS: Clinical use of nitrates. Modern concepts of Cardiovascular disease 68: 37 (1979).
25. Garett Lee et al: Effects of long-term oral administration of Isosorbide Dinitrate on the antianginal response to nitroglycerin. Amer J Cardiol 41: 82 (1978).
26. Goldbarg AJ et al: Antianginal drugs. Postgrad Med J 46: 94 (1979).
27. Reichek N et al: Sustained effects of Nitroglycerin ointment in patients with Angina pectoris. Circulation 50: 348 (1974).
28. Franciosa JA et al: Nitrate therapy for congestive heart failure. JAMA 240: 443 (1978).
29. Franciosa JA and Cohn JN: Sustained hemodynamic effects of nitrates without tolerance in heart failure. Circulation 58 (Suppl 2) 28 (1978).
30. Gray R et al: Hemodynamic and metabolic effects of Isosorbide Dinitrate in chronic congestive heart failure. Am Heart J 90: 346 (1975).

31. Hardarson Th et al: Prolonged salutary effects of Isosorbide Dinitrate and nitroglycerin ointment on regional left ventricular function. Amer J Cardiol 40: 90 (1977).
32. Kovick RB et al: Vasodilator therapy for chronic left ventricular failure. Circulation 53: 322 (1976).
33. Massie B et al: Hemodynamic advantage of combined administration of hydralazine orally and nitrates non parenterally in the vasodilator therapy of chronic heart failure. Amer J Cardiol 40: 794 (1977).
34. Mehta J et al: Nonparenteral combined afterload and preload reduction therapy in congestive heart failure. Clin Cardiol 1: 68 (1978).
35. Williams DO et al: Hemodynamic assessment of oral peripheral vasodilator therapy in chronic congestive heart failure: prolonged effectiveness of Isosorbide Dinitrate. Amer J Cardiol 39: 84 (1977).
36. Rush ML et al: Studies on compensatory reflexes and tolerance to glyceryl trinitrate. Europ J Pharmacol 16: 148 (1971).

Authors' address:
Dr. P. Schlup
Spital Grenchen
CH-2540 Grenchen

Discussion

ABRAMS:

I am not sure that this work is directly related to the explosives industries, but certainly plethysmographic pulse wave evaluations suggest that chronic nitrate exposure leads to changes, in venous return and contraregulation mechanisms, and that with withdrawal of the nitrates on weekends or holidays there is unopposed vasoconstriction. So your hypothesis would be in concert with some of the earlier writings on industrial workers nitrate dependence.

KALTENBACH:

Would you just repeat the dose of isosorbide dinitrate?

SCHLUP:

We used 60 mg ISDN daily in healthy volunteers and 80 mg in patients, both in sustained release formulations.

Hemodynamic and Ventricular Dynamic Investigations of Nitrate Tolerance

W. Niederer, H. D. Bethge, K. Bachmann

Introduction

Tolerance to a drug is present if either an increasing dose is necessary in order to obtain a therapeutic effect or there is no efficacy at all. Normally this tolerance disappears after the treatment is discontinued and develops again during a renewed therapy. It is of decisive importance whether a tolerance exists with regard to a particular single effect of the drug or for the therapeutically desirable overall effect. Self-tolerance is the condition whereby a reduction in efficacy develops for the same substance, whereas cross-tolerance is when another similarly acting substance is ineffective.

In 1888 Stewart (32) reported the phenomenon of a possible nitrate tolerance for the first time in the case of a patient with arterial hypertension. The contributions published on this issue until 1960 reported mainly on withdrawal symptoms in workers in the explosives industry when they were temporarily outside their usual working environment (5, 7, 21, 22, 25, 30). These observations indicate, however, not so much a tolerance as a drug dependence. Although tolerance and drug dependence normally occur simultaneously, one phenomenon alone can become a clinical problem: this is possibly important in the case of the nitrate effect. When higher doses and long-acting nitrates were administered in the mid-1970s, the problem of nitrate tolerance became clinically important because the possibility of effective long-term treatment thereby became questionable.

This issue is rendered all the more topical by the fact that the indications list for nitrates has been extended during recent years, and they are now used for vasodilatation in patients with cardiac insufficiency (9, 16, 29). The results mentioned in the literature concerning nitrate tolerance are contradictory. Some of them speak in favor of a possible tolerance during long-term nitrate therapy in the cases of patients with chronic pulmonary or coronary heart disease (4, 28, 31). The majority of studies, however, prove that administration of nitrates has a steady therapeutic result (3, 6, 8, 11, 14, 15, 17, 20, 23–27, 35) even if tolerance to a single effect may be observed.

The findings for and against nitrate tolerance existing up to now are based on clinical findings such as angina pectoris, exercise tolerance, and nitrate consumption, as well as exercise ECG, arterial blood pressure, and exercise-induced pulmonary hypertension. In addition to these parameters we have examined the function of the left ventricle during exercise under an acute and long-term treatment with isosorbide dinitrate (ISDN).

Case Material

We examined self-tolerance to nitrates in a group of ten coronary patients with an average age of 56. All of them had exercise-induced angina pectoris as well as an ST-segment depression and an angiographically determined stenosis of more than 75% in at least one coronary artery.

65

Methods of Procedure

All patients were without medication for at least 8 days. The examinations took place regularly before breakfast. The exercise tests were carried out with a speed-dependent bicycle ergometer in the supine position until angina pectoris or an ST-segment depression of at least 1 mm became apparent. We recorded heart rate, arterial blood pressure, pulmonary artery pressure, and the pressure in the left ventricle, and angiographically measured the left-ventricular volumes and the ejection fraction. The tests, which were first carried out without medication, both at rest and under stress, were repeated 15 min later after a single administration of 60 mg ISDN.
Subsequently the patients were treated with 60 mg three times a day for an average period of 4 weeks. The last single dose of the long-term treatment was administered 2 h before the control which followed the same protocol. The statistical evaluation of the results was performed according to the paired t-test at the 1% significance level.

Results

The patients' output was 40 ± 21 W over an average of 3 min during the first exercise test, which was performed without any pharmacological influence on the circulation. The ST segments were 2.2 ± 0.7 mm lower. The mean pressure in the pulmonary artery increased from a resting value of 19 ± 4 mmHg to 32 ± 6 mmHg, the filling pressure in the left ventricle rose from 13 ± 3 mmHg to 26 ± 3 mmHg, and the ejection fraction decreased from $67\% \pm 10\%$ to $53\% \pm 12\%$ (Table 1).
After a single dose of 60 mg ISDN the filling pressure in the left ventricle did not increase any further during the ergometry. With a value of 11 ± 5 mmHg it was unchanged from the resting value of 10 ± 4 mmHg. After a 4-week course of ISDN the preload reduction at rest and during ergometry was maintained with values of 11 ± 4 mmHg and 12 ± 4 mmHg respectively (Fig. 1). In accordance with the lasting preload reduction, no ST-segment depression in the ECG or angina pectoris occurred under identical stress conditions in the patients.
The lasting preload reduction under long-term ISDN treatment could also be shown with regard to the pulmonary artery pressure. After administration of a single dose the mean pulmonary artery pressure stayed within the normal range with a value of 16 ± 4 mmHg during ergometry. Even under long-term therapy no stress-related increase could be de-

Table 1. ST-segment depression (ST), mean pulmonary artery pressure ($\overline{PAP}$), left-ventricular end-diastolic pressure (LVEDP) and ejection fraction (EF) in a group of ten coronary patients before therapy. Mean values at rest and during work-induced angina pectoris.

N = 10	Watts	ST↓ (mm)	$\overline{PAP}$ (mmHg)	LVEDP (mmHg)	EF (%)
Rest			19 ± 4	13 ± 3	67 ± 10
Ergo	40 ± 21	2.2 ± 0.7	32 ± 6	26 ± 3	53 ± 12

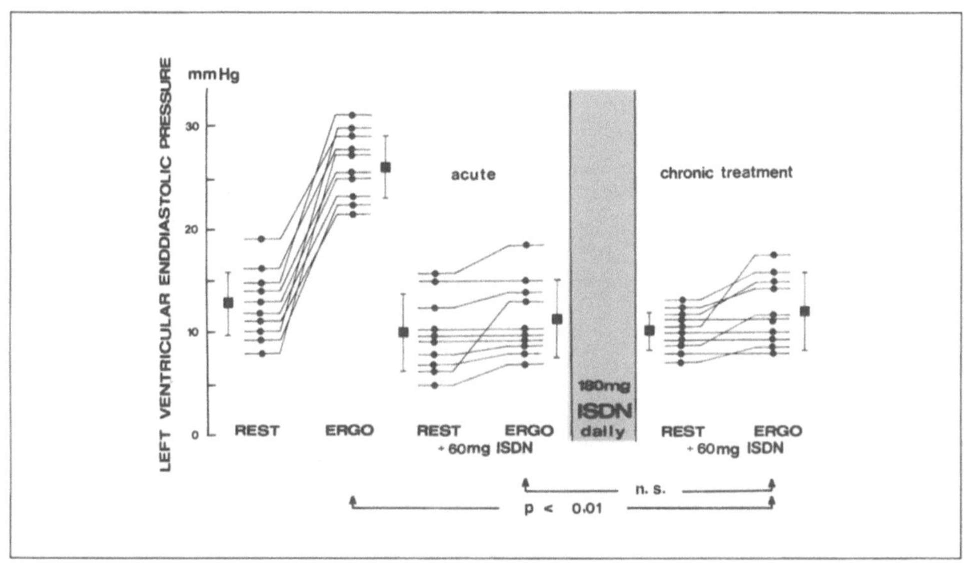

Fig. 1. Left-ventricular enddiastolic pressure before therapy and after acute and chronic treatment with sustained-release isosorbide dinitrate (ISDN). There were no significant changes after the long-term treatment as compared to the single dose. *Ergo,* ergometry.

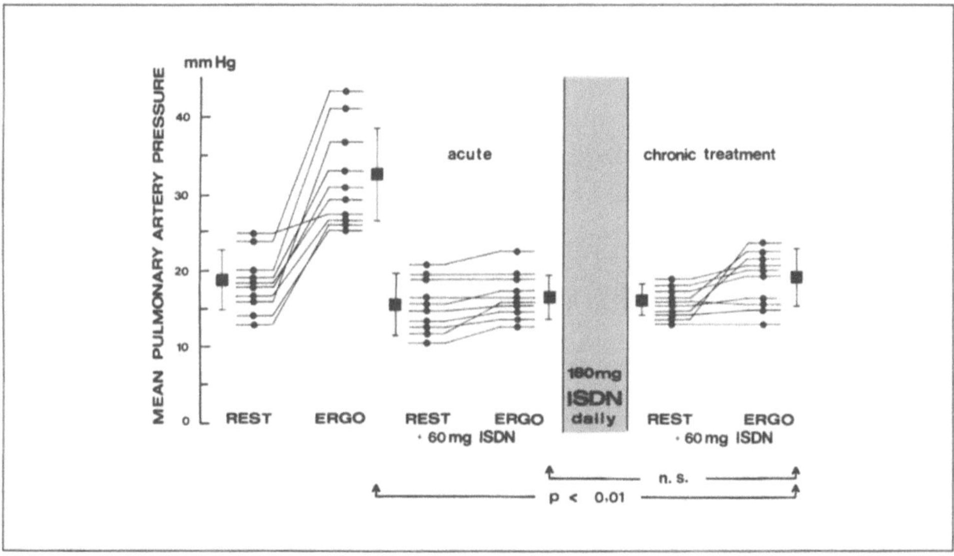

Fig. 2. Mean pulmonary artery pressure before therapy, after a single dose of isosorbide dinitrate (*ISDN*), and during chronic administration for a period of 4 weeks. No significant changes after the chronic treatment as compared to the acute therapy. *Ergo,* ergometry.

tected: the mean pulmonary artery pressure of 19 ± 4 mmHg did not differ significantly after 4 weeks of treatment from the value after a single dose (Fig. 2).

The ejection fraction of the left ventricle decreased without medication from 67% $\pm$ 10%

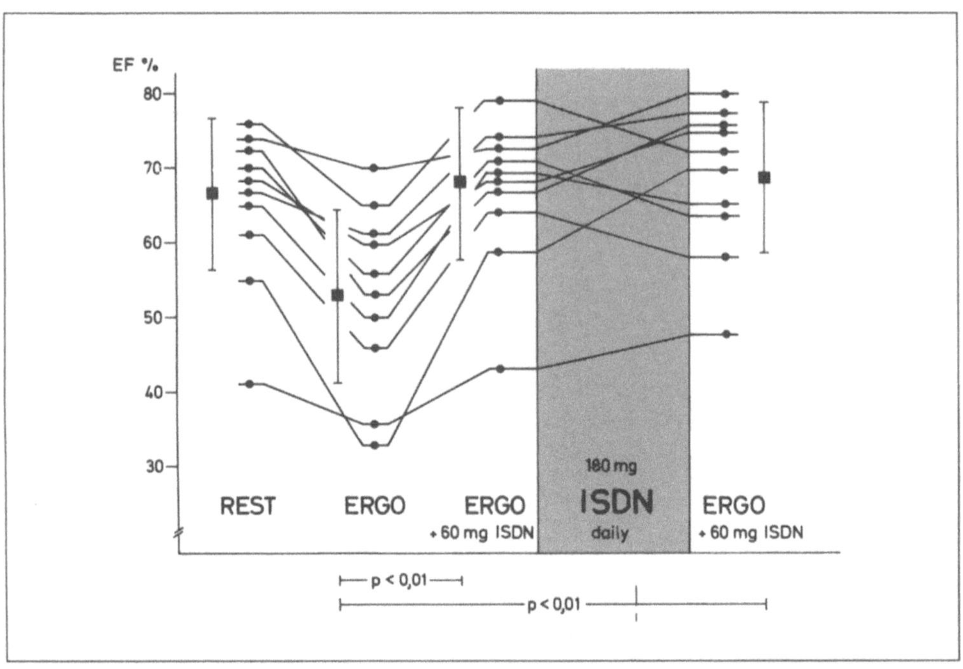

Fig. 3. Ejection fraction before therapy and during acute and chronic administration of sustained-release isosorbide dinitrate (*ISDN*). A single dose of 60 mg ISDN normalizes the exercise-induced degree of the ejection fraction. This beneficial effect was reproducible after chronic treatment. *Ergo*, ergometry.

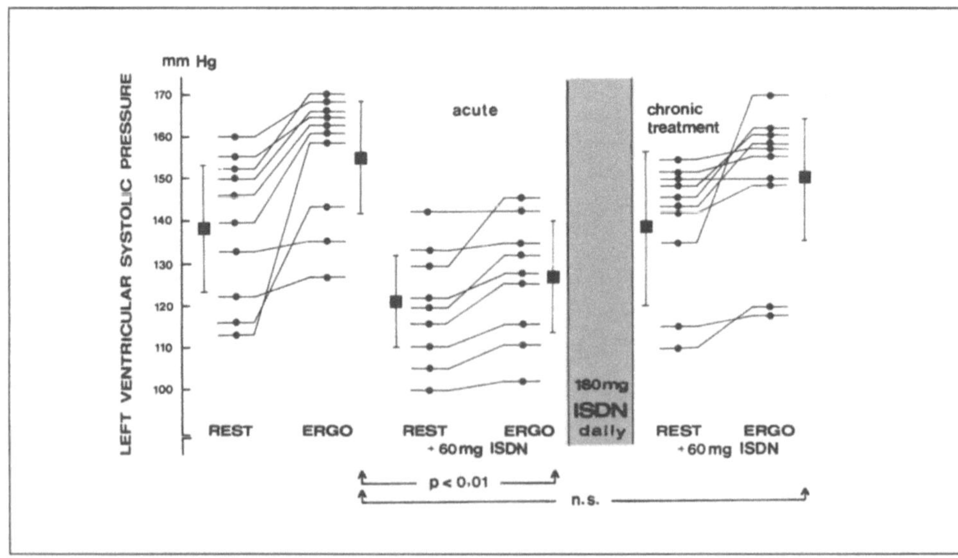

Fig. 4. Left-ventricular systolic pressure during acute and chronic treatment with sustained-release isosorbide dinitrate (*ISDN*). The value after 4 weeks' long-term treatment does not differ significantly from the value before the treatment. *Ergo*, ergometry.

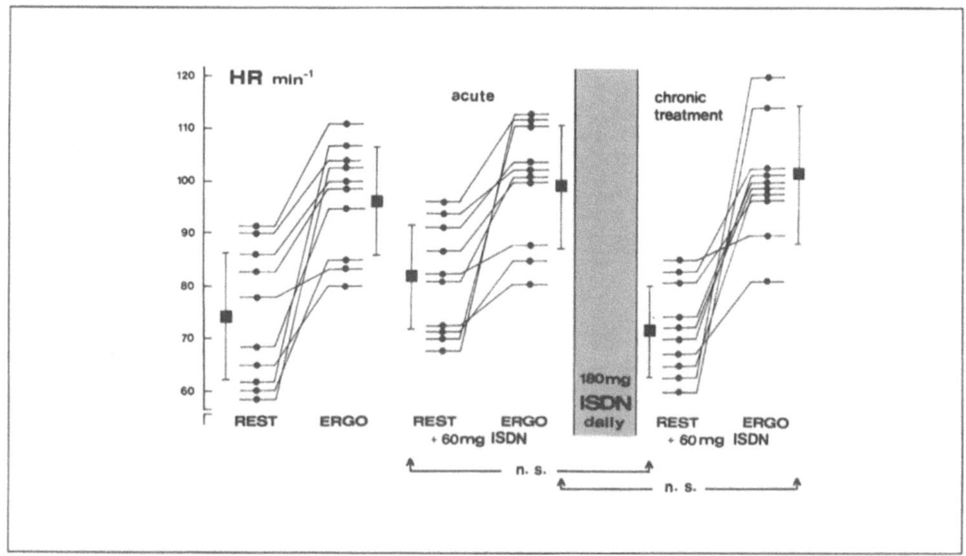

Fig. 5. Heart rate during acute and chronic treatment with isosorbide dinitrate (*ISDN*). No significant changes after long-term medication as compared to the single dose either at rest or during ergometry (*Ergo*).

at rest to 53% ± 12% during ergometry. This decrease in ventricular function was no longer detectable after a single dose of 60 mg ISDN, and the ejection fraction stayed within its normal range with a value of 69% ± 10%. This improvement of ventricular function with an ejection fraction of 60% ± 10% stayed reproducibly detectable even after a long-term treatment of 4 weeks (Fig. 3).

Contrary to the findings of the preload-dependent parameters, a nitrate tolerance affecting the arterial system was determined. Without any pharmacological influence on the circulation we found a stress-induced increase in arterial blood pressure from 139 ± 17 mmHg at rest to 155 ± 15 mmHg. During an acute treatment with 60 mg ISDN, the resting value was 121 ± 13 mmHg, while the stress value was only 127 ± 14 mmHg. After a 4-week treatment the blood pressure at rest was 139 ± 19 mmHg, and rose to 155 ± 17 mmHg again when the patients underwent ergometry. The blood pressure at rest as well as under stress thus did not differ from the initial values after chronic nitrate therapy (Fig. 4).

The heart rate at rest increased from 74 ± 13 to 82 ± 11 beats/min after a single dose of 60 mg ISDN, but decreased to 72 ± 9 beats/min during chronic treatment and was thus no longer different from the initial values. The values under stress remained almost identical at 96 ± 11 without medication, 99 ± 12 after a single dose, and 101 ± 15 during chronic treatment (Fig. 5).

Figures 6–8 show the ECG leads V_4, V_5, and V_6, as well as the diastolic pressure in the left ventricle, in patients with one-vessel, two-vessel, or three-vessel disease during exercise with the bicycle ergometer. In the case of angina pectoris, an ischemic ST-segment depression appeared combined with a pathological increase in the filling pressure in the left ventricle if the circulation was not influenced pharmacologically. An identical stress was tolerated without angina pectoris and with an uneventful ECG and a normal end-

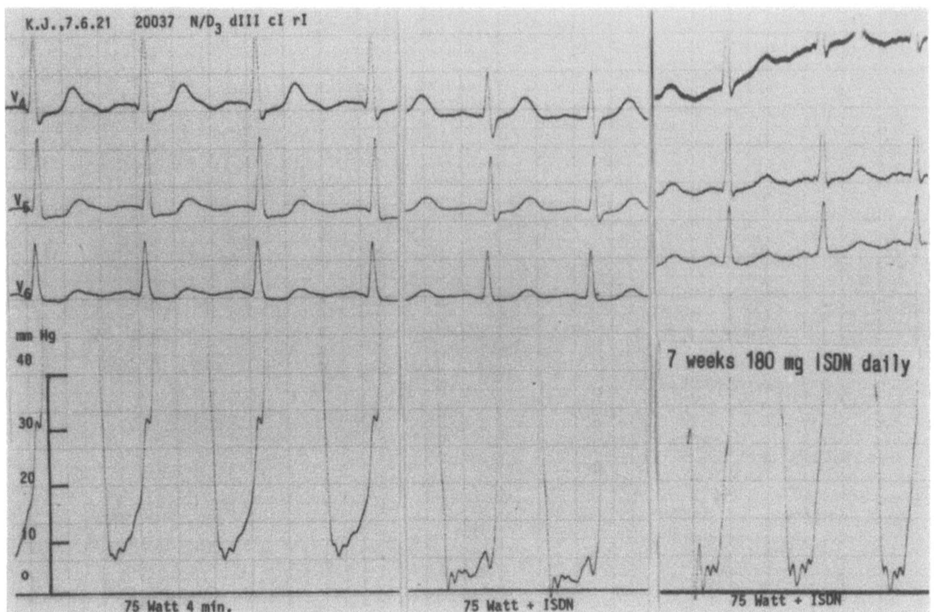

Fig. 6. ST-segment depression (V₅, V₆) and increased left-ventricular filling pressure during exercise at 75 W in a 60-year-old man with one-vessel disease. After a single dose of 60 mg and after long-term treatment with isosorbide dinitrate (*ISDN*), the left-ventricular filling pressure is normalized during identical exercise.

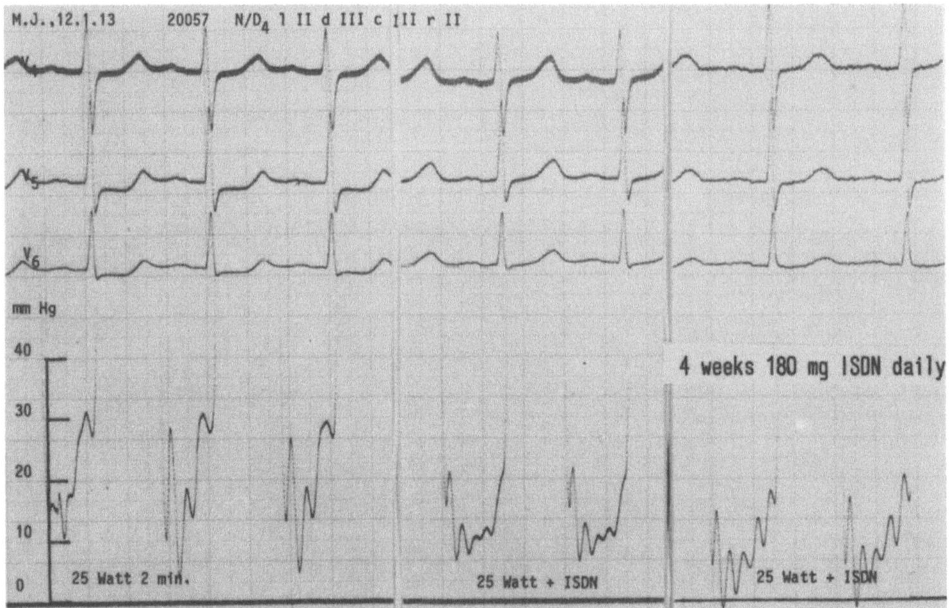

Fig. 7. ST-segment depression and increased left-ventricular filling pressure during exercise at 25 W in a 69-year-old patient with two-vessel disease. After a single dose and after long-term treatment with isosorbide dinitrate (*ISDN*) over 4 weeks the ECG and the left-ventricular enddiastolic pressure are normalized.

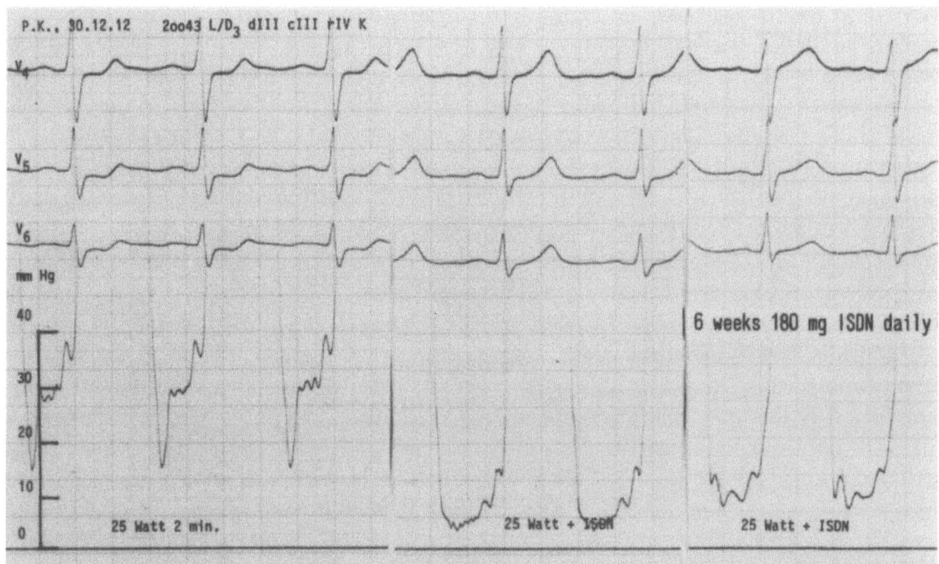

Fig. 8. ST-segment depression and by 30 mmHg increased left-ventricular filling pressure during exercise at 25 W in a 69-year-old patient with three vessel disease. Not only after a single dose but also after long-term treatment with isosorbide dinitrate (*ISDN*) over 6 weeks the ECG and the left-ventricular filling pressure are normalized.

diastolic pressure in the left ventricle after a single dose of 60 mg ISDN under chronic nitrate therapy.

Discussion

During acute treatment with 40 mg ISDN in sustained-release form, as well as with 40 mg normal ISDN, a highly significant decrease in the ST-segment depression could be seen in the stress ECG. The maximum decrease in ischemia was reached in the 4th h (18). A significant decrease in the systolic and diastolic blood pressure, as well as in the pulmonary artery pressure, at rest and during stress, was also detected for longer than 4 h after a single administration of 40 mg ISDN (2, 36). The improvement in stress tolerance under the efficacy of ISDN in capsule form also lasted up to 6 h after the administration of the drug (24). These findings, which were compiled after the acute administration of the drug, make long-term oral therapy with a dosage in sustained-release form seem reasonable if an average duration of effect of 4 h is taken as a basis. The observation that formerly increasing nitrate doses were necessary for the chronic treatment of arterial hypertension and that at the beginning of such treatment headache, nausea, and dizziness appeared but disappeared again after some days (12, 19, 33), led however to the supposition that a tolerance could develop in the case of chronic nitrate treatment. On the other hand, no tolerance with regard to the therapeutic effect was detected in spite of a subsidence of the cerebral vasodilatation (1). Danahy and Aronow observed the same phenomenon (13). In spite of a lasting improvement in the maximum stress tolerance, and a

71

decrease in the ST-segment depression and in symptoms, the effect of nitrates on blood pressure and heart rate was weakened under long-term therapy. These findings, as well as the decrease in headaches, indicate a partial tolerance under chronic ISDN therapy. Our results show a similar reaction with regard to the arterial blood pressure: while it increased from 139 mmHg at rest to 155 mmHg under stress before the ISDN treatment, it was 121 mmHg at rest and rose to only 127 mmHg under stress during bicycle ergometry after acute treatment with ISDN. After long-term treatment the arterial stress blood pressure increased to 155 mmHg again and was thus not different from the initial value when the circulation was not pharmacologically influenced.

Parker (28) also observed a self- and cross-tolerance affecting the arterial blood pressure and the heart rate in spite of a high plasma concentration under long-term therapy with ISDN, although the stress tolerance in comparison with a placebo was significantly better for at least 2 h after administration of the drug. This lasting improvement in symptoms in spite of a partial tolerance with regard to the arterial blood pressure and the heart rate can be explained by the fact that a reduction of the preload also continues under long-term therapy. In our patients, the filling pressure in the left ventricle did not increase any further after a single dose of 60 mg ISDN during ergometry, and it remained constant at 11 mmHg compared with the resting value of 10 mmHg. Even after 4 weeks of ISDN treatment the normalization of the enddiastolic pressure in the left ventricle at rest and during ergometry was maintained at 11–12 mmHg. This lasting preload decrease which could also be recognized by the fact that there was no ST-segment depression or angina pectoris in any of the patients, was also proved by means of pulmonary artery pressure. After 4 weeks of treatment the mean stress pressure in the pulmonary artery was, at a level of 19 mmHg, not significantly different from the value after the first single dose. No cross-tolerance could be detected after an acute administration of nitroglycerin with regard to an unchanged good maximum stress, stress duration, and maximal oxygen absorption under equally high long-term doses of ISDN (120 mg/day). As the lasting decrease in the ST-segment depression under chronic ISDN therapy did not lead to a further reduction of the ST segment after the acute administration of nitroglycerin, a self-tolerance for ISDN could not be detected (23). Among patients suffering from left-ventricular insufficiency a self-tolerance could not be found under therapy with 160 mg of ISDN either. In comparison to placebo a lasting vasodilatation with correspondingly improved clinical symptoms was manifest after 3 months of treatment (15).

These findings are contrary to the results of Blasini et al. (4), who found a significant dose-dependent decrease in blood pressure, an increase in heart rate, and a reduction of the ST segment when they administered long-acting ISDN in single doses of 20, 40, and 60 mg. They were, however, not able to detect any effect on either the parameters mentioned or the frequency of angina pectoris attacks and the nitrate consumption under long-term treatment with the same doses of ISDN administered three times a day.

As the acute efficacy is greatest in the 3rd h, the control examinations were also performed in the 3rd h after the last administration of drug or placebo during long-term therapy. Parker (28) found that the stress tolerance under chronic nitrate therapy was, in comparison to the placebo, significantly higher only up to the 2nd h after administration. Our examinations, which proved a continuously lasting preload reduction during chronic ISDN therapy, were performed 15 min after ISDN administration. It is possible that Blasini's negative findings are due to a decrease in the efficacy time of ISDN in long-term treatment. In contrast to Parker's (28) findings there are, however, the results of Lee (24), who found a lasting improvement in the maximum stress and a decrease in ST-segment depression up to 6 h after drug administration under chronic ISDN treatment.

In conclusion, our results confirm the observation that acute nitrate efficacy is no longer detectable with regard to the resting and stress blood pressure after long-term treatment with ISDN. On the other hand, however, they show that after treatment with 180 mg ISDN per day over an average period of 4 weeks the influence on the preload-dependent parameters remains unaltered. The phenomenon of self-tolerance can thus be seen in the arterial blood pressure but not in the therapeutically decisive preload.

The question whether the preload reduction under long-term nitrate therapy does not last as long as with acute administration can only be answered after further study.

References

1. Abrams J: Nitrate tolerance and dependence. Amer Heart J 99: 113 (1980).
2. Bachmann K, Zerzawy R und Fleischer H: Beurteilung von Nitropräparaten bei Koronarkranken im Alltag mittels Telemetrie. In: Rudolph W und Siegenthaler W (Hrsgb): Nitrate. Wirkung auf Herz und Kreislauf. Urban & Schwarzenberg, München-Berlin-Wien 1976.
3. Becker HJ, Walden G, Kaltenbach M: Gibt es eine „Tachyphylaxie" beziehungsweise Gewöhnung bei der Behandlung der Angina pectoris mit Nitrokörpern. Verh dtsch Ges inn Med 82: 1208 (1976).
4. Blasini R, Brügmann U, Mannes A, Froer KL, Hall D und Rudolph W: Wirksamkeit von Isosorbiddinitrat in retardierter Form bei Langzeitbehandlung. Herz 5: 298 (1980).
5. Bright GE: The effects of nitroglycerin on those engaged in its manufacture. JAMA 62: 201 (1914).
6. Brunner D, Weisbrod J, Meshulam N, Margulis S: Langzeitwirkung und Dauertherapie mit kutan appliziertem Isosorbiddinitrat. Münch med Wschr 122: 801 (1980).
7. Carmichael P and Lieben J: Sudden death in explosives workers. Arch Environ Health 7: 50 (1963).
8. Chandraratna PAN, Langevin E, O'Dell R, Rubinstein C, and San Pedro S: Use of nitroglycerin ointment in congestive heart failure. Cardiology 63: 337 (1978).
9. Chatterjee K, Massie B, Rubin S, Gelberg H, Brundage BH, and Ports TA: Long-term outpatient vasodilator therapy of congestive heart failure. Consideration of agents at rest and during exercise. Am J Med 65: 134 (1978).
10. Cohn JN, Mathew KJ, Franciosa JA, and Snow JA: Chronic vasodilator therapy in the management of cardiogenic shock and intractable left ventricular failure. Ann Intern Med 81: 177 (1974).
11. Cole SL and Kaye H: Antianginal effects of oral, controlled-release nitroglycerin in patients with coronary artery disease: Double-blind randomized, multiple cross-over study. Clin Res 23: 177 (1975).
12. Crandall LA, Leake CD, Loevenhart AS, and Muehlberger CW: Acquired tolerance to and cross tolerance between the nitrous and nitric acid esters and sodium nitrite in man. J Pharmacol Exp Ther 41: 103 (1931).
13. Danahy DT, and Aronow WS: Hemodynamics and antianginal effects of high dose oral isosorbide dinitrate after chronic use. Circulation 56: 205 (1977).
14. Davidov MF and Mroczek WJ: The effect of sustained release nitroglycerine capsules on anginal frequency and exercise capacity. Angiology 28: 181 (1977).
15. Franciosa JA and Cohn JN: Sustained hemodynamic effects of nitrates without tolerance in heart failure. Circulation 58: (Suppl. 2) 28 (1978).
16. Franciosa SA, Nordstrom LA and Cohn JN: Nitrate therapy for congestive heart failure. JAMA 240: 443 (1978).
17. Gray R, Vyden J, Chatterjee K, Ganz W, Forrester JS, and Swan HJC: Hemodynamic and metabolic effects of isosorbide dinitrate in chronic congestive heart failure. Am Heart J 90: 346 (1975).

18. Hennermann KH, Becker HJ, und Kaltenbach M: Vergleich der Wirkungsdauer und Intensität oral applizierter Einzeldosen von 40 mg isoket® bzw. isoket® retard im Belastungs-EKG bei Patienten mit koronarer Herzkrankheit. In: Rudolph W und Schrey A (Hrsgb): Nitrate II. Wirkung auf Herz und Kreislauf. 2. Nitrat-Symposium Berlin. Urban & Schwarzenberg, München-Wien-Baltimore 1980.

19. Horwitz LD, Herman MV, Corlin R: Clinical Response to Nitroglycerin as a Diagnostic Test for Coronary Artery Disease. Amer J Cardiol 29: 149 (1972).

20. Kovic RB, Tillisch JH, Berens SC, Bramowitz AD, and Shine KI: Vasodilator therapy for chronic left ventricular failure. Circulation 53: 322 (1976).

21. Laws GC: The effects of nitroglycerin upon those who manufacture it. JAMA 31 (1898).

22. Laws CE: Nitroglycerin head. JAMA 54: 793 (1910).

23. Lee G, Mason DT, and DeMaria AN: Effects of long-term oral administration of isosorbide dinitrate on the antianginal response to nitroglycerin. Absence of nitrate cross-tolerance and self-tolerance shown by exercise testing. Am J Cardiol 41: 82 (1978).

24. Lee G, Mason DT, Amsterdam EA, Miller RR, and DeMaria AN: Angianginal efficacy of oral therapy with isosorbide dinitrate capsules. Chest 73: 327 (1978).

25. Lund RP, Haggendahl J, and Johnsson G: Withdrawal symptoms in workers exposed to nitroglycerine. Br J Ind Med 25: 136 (1968).

26. Massie B, Chatterjee K, Werner J, Greenberg B, Hart R, and Parmley WW: Hemodynamic advantage of combined administration of hydralazine orally and nitrates nonparenterally in the vasodilator therapy of chronic heart failure. Am J Cardiol 40: 794 (1977).

27. Mehta J, Pepine CJ, and Conti CR: Nonparenteral combined afterload and preload reduction therapy in congestive heart failure. Clin Cardiol 1: 68 (1978).

28. Parker JO, Thadani U: Tolerance to the circulatory and clinical effects of nitrates. Abstract. In: Lichtlen PR, Engel AJ, Schrey A, Swan HJC (ed): Nitrates III. Springer Verlag, Berlin-Heidelberg-New York 1981.

29. Pierpont LL, Cohn JN, and Franciosa JA: Combined oral hydralazine-nitrate therapy in left ventricular failure. Chest 73: 8 (1978).

30. Schwartz AM: The cause, relief and prevention of headaches arising from contact with dynamite. N Engl J Med 235: 651 (1946).

31. Schüren KP und Macha HN: Isosorbiddinitrate bei chronischem Cor pulmonale. Münch Med Wschr 103: 777 (1978).

32. Stewart DD: Remarkable tolerance to nitroglycerin. Philadelphia Polyclinic, p 172 (1888).

33. Stewart DD: Tolerance to nitroglycerin. JAMA 44: 1678 (1905).

34 Thadani U, Manyari D, Parker JO, Fung H: Tolerance to the circulatory effects of oral isosorbide dinitrate. Rate of development and cross-tolerance to glyceryl trinitrate. Circulation 61: 526 (1980).

35. Winsor W and Berger HJ: Oral nitroglycerin as a prophylactic antianginal drug: Clinical, physiologic and statistical evidence of efficacy based on a threephase experimental design. Am Heart J 90: 611 (1975).

36. Zerzawy R und Bachmann K: Langzeitwirkung von 40 mg Isosorbiddinitrat. Plasmaspiegel und Hämodynamik in Ruhe und während Ergometrie im Liegen und Sitzen. In: Rudolph W und Schrey A (eds.): Nitrate II. Wirkung auf Herz und Kreislauf. 2. Nitrat-Symposium Berlin. Urban & Schwarzenberg, München-Wien-Baltimore 1980.

Authors' address:
Priv.-Doz. Dr. W. Niederer
Medizinische Poliklinik der
Universität Erlangen-Nürnberg
Östliche Stadtmauerstr. 29
8520 Erlangen

Discussion

KALTENBACH:

I am very impressed by the considerable amount of data from so many patients. If there was tolerance only to the blood pressure reaction, this would be in contrast to Dr. Tauchert's findings. Maybe the difference is not so large, if we assume that the findings of Dr. Tauchert reflect pulmonary artery pressure but not necessarily left ventricular pressure.

FRANCIOSA:

Our experience reagarding systolic blood pressure during exercise is exactly like yours. All the changes we saw were on the pulmonary wedge pressure. The systolic arterial pressure was not affected, either acutely or chronically by single doses of isosorbide dinitrate during exercise.

ABRAMS:

I would like to compliment you on this very elegant study. We associate the parameters measured by you with ischemia-induced left ventricular dysfunction, and you have clinical correlates in terms of response that make sense in angina patients. This goes along with our clinical impressions of a lot of data we have heard about today, and I think sometimes we ought to remember that we are dealing with patients and control of patients' symptoms and that this kind of study looks at very clear pathophysiologic changes related to symptoms and to angina and shows, at least in this small group, that tolerance is not present, on the one hands, and that on the other, nitrates are very useful for patients with ischemia of the left ventricle.

DEMARIA:

Were exercises conduced in supine position and were ventriculographies done during exercise just afterwards and in which projection? Did you have problems with volume measurements during respiration?

NIEDERER:

The patients were pedaling the bicycle in supine position while the ventriculograms were performed in 3° AOP, without any problems with respiration.

FOX:

The four examples after treatment with ISDN showed no ST-segment changes. I am not sure whether one can assume that the failure of rise of left-ventricular enddiastolic pressure is related to venous adaptation, rather than in some way to the ISDN, as preventing ischaemia. Normally one would expect a rise in left-ventricular enddiastolic pressure during ischaemia, and I don't know whether we can actually dissect how the drug has worked.

BACHMANN:

May I comment in the place of Dr. Niederer. I think we all agree that venous dilatation and reduction in preload are the primary effects of nitrates, and what we didn't mention is that in the same group of ten patients we made a study on the tilting table with arterial blood pressure measurements and we came to the conclusion that in the acute treatment there was orthostatic hypotension in every patient, and when we repeated tilting table tests after 4 weeks, the blood pressure regulation was completely normalized. With these results in mind concluded, that there is tolerance due to adaptation of the arterial system in patients after four weeks of ISDN treatment, but not in the venous system, since as far as left ventricular preload is concerned, we found the same effects as compared to acute treatment. This may explain why the pressure rate product is not a dominant factor in assessing the effect of nitrates, because by adaptation of the arterial pressure and with no change in heart rate during chronic treatment no significant reduction in pressure/rate product can be expected.

ABRAMS:

We are all aware that there is now some suggestive work showing that even in exercise-induced angina a component of coronary vasal motor tone alteration may be involved. In Dr. Niederer's patients, an improvement of the ejection fraction has been found. In addition, one could suggest that increased compliance of the ischemic ventricle, i.e. the pressure volume loop may well have been improved with nitrates, whether this was due to preload reduction or to improvement of subendocardial regional blood flow. But we have to be careful in talking about the venous versus the arterial effects in so simplified terms.

FRANCIOSA:

I just wanted to speculate that the improved ejection fraction was perhaps due to the elevated stroke volume, and that is why the systolic blood pressure went down during exercise. This study has indeed, not shown any tolerance to the effect of nitrates.

KOBER:

We heard that there may be some tolerance or counterregulation on the arterial side and the investigations of Needleman showed that there is tolerance in aortic strips in in-vitro experiments. On the other hand, Dr. Schlup has not found tolerance in the arterial bed. As regards the venous bed, there were some indications of tolerance in older studies by Mason. In most studies, no tolerance regarding haemodynamic parameters has been found. Are there any data available on in-vitro experiments with vein strips?

FUNG:

I don't know about venous in-vitro data. The methodology on the venous side is much more difficult than on the arterial side.

DEMARIA:

I would like to inform about a new development for the Apollo space program, which uses ultrasound. Thus, venous tone and arterial tone can be measured. Perhaps the questions just raised could be answered with this method.

Treatment of Congestive Heart Failure with Vasodilators: Comparison of Acute and Long-Term Effects of Various Agents

G. F. Hauf, P. Bubenheimer, and H. Roskamm

Introduction

Uncontestedly vasodilators, independent of their primary site of action, initially exert a favorable effect in patients with acute or chronic congestive and forward heart failure. This has been documented by hemodynamic as well as clinical findings. However the extent to which such treatment results in a sustained improvement of hemodynamics, subjective complaints, or even prognosis remains controversial.

Numerous studies carried out in the recent past suggest that reliable predictions generally regarding the success of long-term therapy are not possible. We therefore attempted to contribute toward a clarification of the following questions:

1. To what extent does the initial acute administration of a vasodilator affect hemodynamics in patients with severe congestive heart failure?
2. Can a change in cardiovascular conditions still be achieved even after a 16-h drug-free interval following long-term maintenance vasodilator therapy?
3. Can a renewed acute administration of the vasodilator exert a hemodynamic effect following a 16-h drug-free interval subsequent to longer-term vasodilator therapy? If yes, are the same improvements achieved as during the initial acute application?
4. With regard to the aforementioned questions, are there differences discernible among vasodilators with different sites of action?

As a representative of drugs which predominantly reduce preload, isosorbide dinitrate (ISDN) in sustained-release form was used; as a representative of agents which equally reduce preload and afterload we selected prazosin; and as a substance that predominantly diminishes afterload, we employed dihydralazine.

Table 1. Characteristics of patient groups on the basis of clinical parameters obtained prior to the study. Roentgenographic findings: absolute heart volume (HV), heart volume relative to body weight (HV/kg); echocardiographic findings: left-ventricular enddiastolic diameter (ED), shortening fraction (SF), coronary heart disease (CHD), and cardiomyopathy (CMP)

	Age (years)	Diagnosis	HV (ml)	HV/kg (ml/kg)	ED (mm)	SF
Total (N·= 16)	51.1 (43–65)	CHD 6 CMP 10	1485	18.5	69.8 (N = 13)	0.14 (N = 13)
ISDN (N = 4)	52.6 (43–65)	CHD 2 CMP 2	1416	16.8	70 (N = 3)	0.14 (N = 3)
Prazosin (N = 5)	50.8 (47–55)	CHD 2 CMP 3	1365	18.8	68.2 (N = 5)	0.15 (N = 5)
Dihydralazine (N = 7)	50.1 (45–58)	CHD 2 CMP 5	1674	20.0	71.2 (N = 5)	0.13 (N = 5)

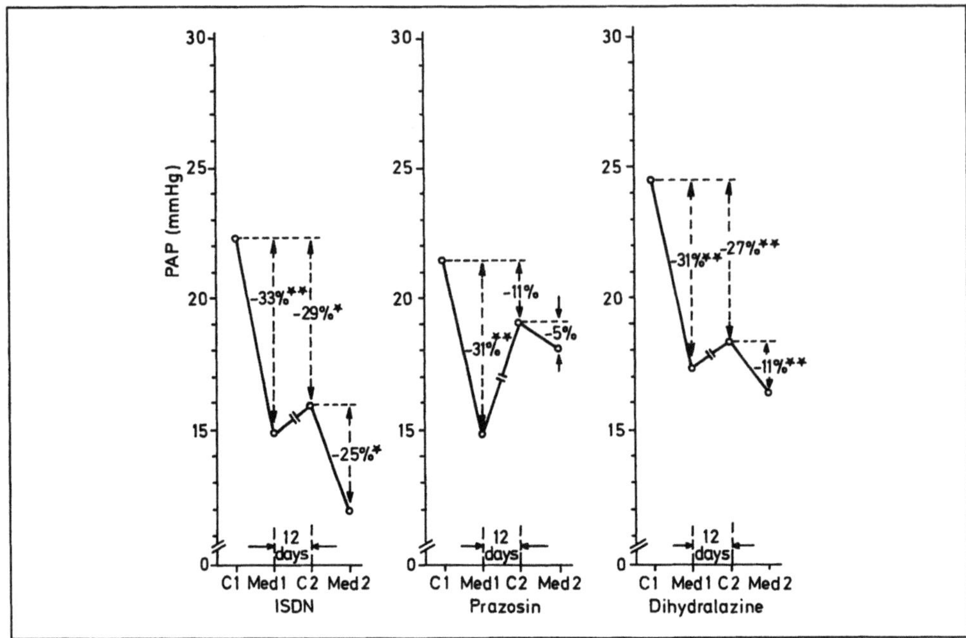

Fig. 1. Enddiastolic pulmonary artery pressure (*PAP*) before vasodilator administration (*C 1*), following initial vasodilator administration (*Med 1*), at follow-up after a 12-day course of treatment and a 16-h drug-free interval (*C 2*), and on renewed acute administration of the vasodilator (*Med 2*). *ISDN*, isosorbide dinitrate 20 mg three times a day (N = 4); *Prazosin*, prazosin 2 mg three times a day (N = 5); *Dihydralazine*, dihydralazine 75 mg three times a day (N = 7). * $p < 0.05$; ** $p < 0.01$.

Patient Characteristics

The hemodynamic response to an initial administration of vasodilators was studied in conjuction with the response to chronic administration of a given agent in 16 male patients with severe congestive heart failure (Table 1). The mean age was 51.1 years. The severity of the clinical impression is characterized by both roentgenographic heart volume (1485 ml absolute, 18.5 ml/kg body wt) and echocardiographic left-ventricular enddiastolic diameter (69.8 mm), as well as shortening fraction (0.14). Etiologically, heart failure was attributable to either a large previous myocardial infarction or congestive cardiomyopathy.

In accordance with our objective of comparing various vasodilators, three subgroups were formed to investigate acute and long-term effects:

1. ISDN group (N = 4); no previous nitrate therapy
2. Prazosin group (N = 5); no previous prazosin therapy
3. Hydralazine group (N = 7); no previous hydralazine therapy.

Methods

The current drug regimen was maintained for at least 7 days. This phase was followed by a 16-h drug-free interval. Subsequently, following determination of the baseline para-

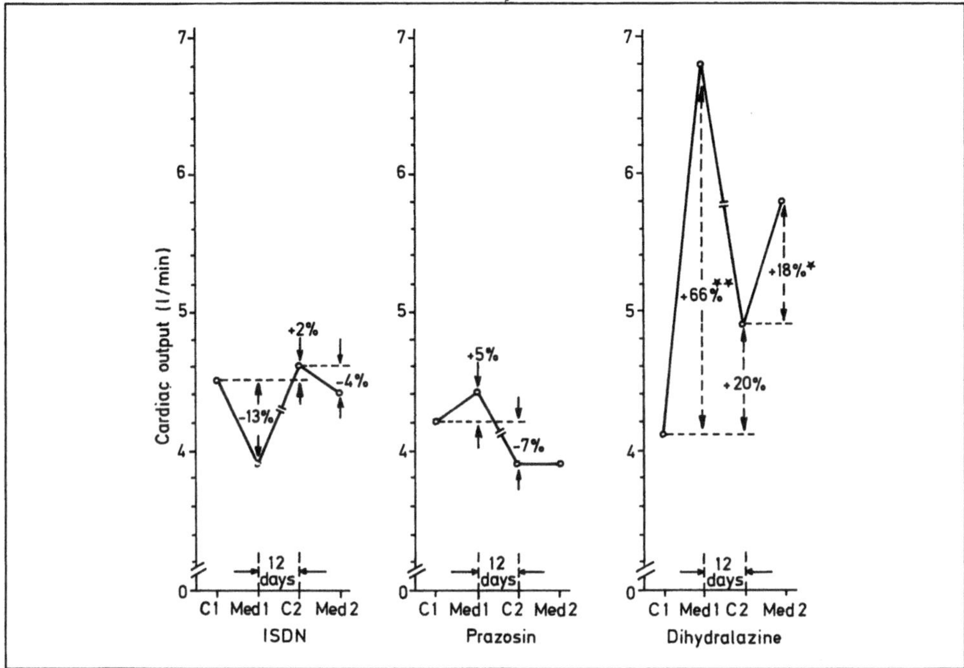

Fig. 2. Cardiac output before vasodilator administration (*C 1*), following initial vasodilator administration (*Med 1*), at follow-up after a 12-day course of treatment and a 16-h drug-free interval (*C 2*), and on renewed acute administration of the vasodilator (*Med 2*). *ISDN,* isosorbide dinitrate 20 mg three times a day (N = 4); *Prazosin,* prazosin 2 mg three times a day (N = 5); *Dihydralazine,* dihydralazine 75 mg three times a day (N = 7). $*p < 0.05$; $**p < 0.01$.

meters, ISDN 40 mg in sustained-release form (Isoket retard 40) orally in conjunction with ISDN 5 mg (Isoket) sublingually, prazosin 2 mg (Minipress) or dihydralazine 75 mg (Nepresol) was administered to the three respective subgroups. During this phase of the investigation, continuous hemodynamic monitoring of the patients was carried out by means of right-heart, flow-directed catheterization.

After the effect of the vasodilator had been established, the ongoing therapy was continued together with the acutely administered agent at dosages of 20 mg ISDN in sustained-release form three times a day, 2 mg prazosin three times a day, and 75 mg dihydralazine three times a day. This regimen was maintained without interruption for 12 days. Another 16-h drug-free interval followed, after which the second phase of hemodynamic monitoring was carried out to determine again the acute effect of the vasodilator administered during the 12-day period. Again, the following doses were used: ISDN sustained-release 40 mg in conjunction with ISDN 5 mg, prazosin 2 mg, or dihydralazine 75 mg.

Results

In Figs. 1–3, the abscissae represent time and the ordinates the corresponding absolute values. Each subgroup is shown separately.

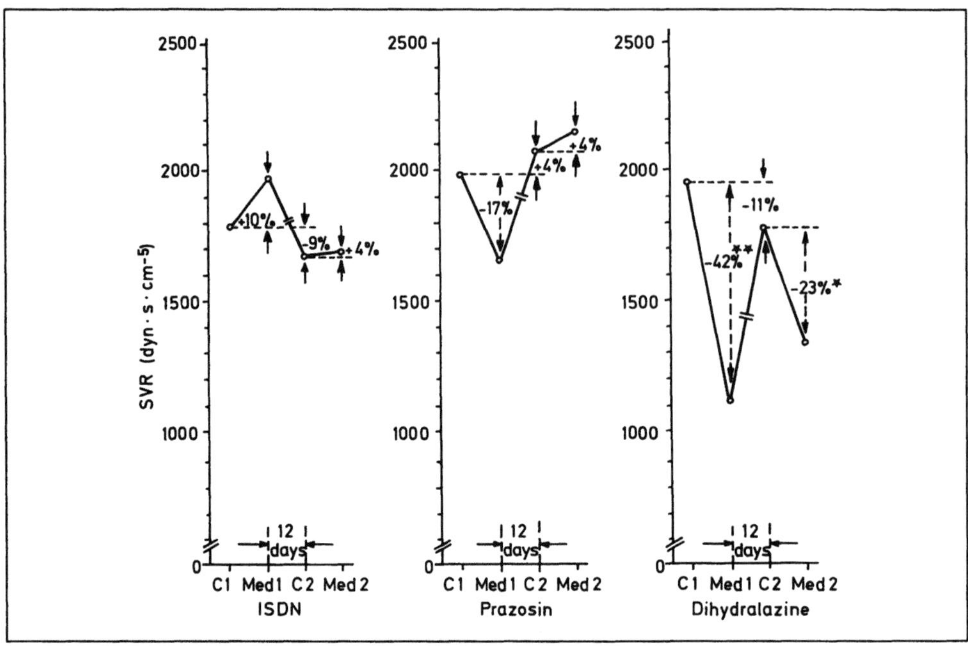

Fig. 3. Systemic vascular resistance (*SVR*) before vasodilator administration (*C 1*), following initial vasodilator administration (*Med 1*), at follow-up after a 12-day course of treatment and a 16-h drug-free interval (*C 2*), and on renewed acute administration of the vasodilator (*Med 2*). *ISDN*, isosorbide dinitrate 20 mg three times a day (N = 4); *Prazosin*, prazosin 2 mg three times a day (N = 5); *Dihydralazine*, dihydralazine 75 mg three times a day (N = 7). * $p < 0.05$; ** $p < 0.01$.

Changes in Enddiastolic Pulmonary Artery Pressure *ISDN Group.* The hemodynamic studies prior to the onset of long-term vasodilator therapy showed an enddiast. Pulmonary artery pressure of 22.4 mmHg. The first acute administration of ISDN was associated with a significant decline in pressure to 15 mmHg (corresponding to −33%). The second hemodynamic monitoring, which was carried out after a 16-h drug-free interval following 12 days of low-dose (20 mg ISDN three times a day) vasodilator therapy, disclosed an enddiast. pulmonary artery pressure of 16 mmHg (corresponding to −29%).
The repeated acute administration of ISDN resulted in a further significant decline in enddiast. pulmonary artery pressure to 12 mmHg (corresponding to −25%).

Prazosin Group. The initial value of enddiastolic pulmonary artery pressure in this group of patients was 21.6 mmHg. The first acute administration of prazosin 2 mg yielded a significant reduction to 15 mmHg (−31%). The follow-up investigation after 12 days showed a slight, insignificant reduction in pressure (19.2 mmHg or −11%). The repeated acute administration of prazosin 2 mg caused no additional changes (18.2 mmHg or −5%, NS).
Dihydralazine Group. The baseline value of enddiastolic pulmonary artery pressure before dihydralazine therapy was 24.9 mmHg. The acute administration of dihydralazine 75 mg caused a significant decline to 17.3 mmHg (−31%). The follow-up value showed a persistence in the pressure reduction, with an enddiast. pulmonary artery pressure of 18.3

mmHg (or –27%). The renewed acute administration of dihydralazine yielded a further significant decrease in pressure to 16.3 mmHg (or –11%).

Changes in Cardiac Output

ISDN Group. After the initial administration of ISDN, cardiac output decreased from 4.5 l/min to 3.9 l/min (or –13%). The follow-up measurement, 4.6 l/min, was comparable to the first determination (+2%). The additional acute administration also did not affect cardiac output (4.4 l/min or –4%).

Prazosin Group. The initial administration of prazosin resulted in a cardiac output of 4.4 l/min (or +5%), which represented virtually no change in relation to the baseline value, 4.2 l/min. The follow-up investigation yielded a value of 3.9 l/min, a minimal insignificant reduction of –7%. Acute administration now also failed to cause any change in cardiac output.

Dihydralazine Group. With an initial cardiac output of 4.1 l/min, the first administration of the vasodilator produced a significant (+ 66%) increase to 6.8 l/min. After a 12-day course of dihydralazine, cardiac output remained increased to 4.9 l/min (+ 20%), a value which was not significantly different from baseline values, however. The renewed administration of dihydralazine again caused a significant increase in cardiac output to 5.8 l/min (or + 18%).

Changes in Systemic Vascular Resistance

ISDN Group. Systemic vascular resistance prior to the initiation of vasodilator therapy was 1794 dyn · sec · cm^{-5}. Following acute application of ISDN, it increased by 10% (1980 dyn · sec · cm^{-5}). The follow-up measurement after 12 days showed that systemic vascular resistance had fallen by –9% (1638 dyn · sec · cm^{-5}). The renewed acute application of ISDN however, resulted in a slight increase in resistance by + 4% (1965 dyn · sec · cm^{-5}).

Prazosin Group. With a baseline value of 1995 dyn · sec · cm^{-5}, the acute application resulted in a –17% change in systemic vascular resistance, a change which was not significant, however (1660 dyn · sec · cm^{-5}). The subsequent follow-up yielded a value comparable to the baseline measurement (2071 dyn · sec · cm^{-5}). The renewed administration of prazosin was virtually without any effect (2145 dyn · sec · cm^{-5} or + 4%).

Dihydralazine Group. The initial administration of dihydralazine 75 mg yielded a significant (–42%) reduction in resistance (1119 dyn · sec · cm^{-5}) from the baseline value of 1935 dyn · sec · cm^{-5}. Even after 12 days of medication a –11% reduction was found (1731 dyn · sec · cm^{-5}), which was not significant, however. The renewed acute administration of dihydralazine again produced a significant (–23%) reduction (1328 dyn · sec · cm^{-5}) compared to the second control value.

Table 2. Characteristics of patient group having undergone previous long-term vasodilator therapy. Roentgenographic findings: absolute heart volume (HV), heart volume relative to body weight (HV/kg); echocardiographic findings: left-ventricular enddiastolic diameter (ED), shortening fraction (SF), coronary heart disease (CHD), cardiomyopathy (CMP)

	Age (years)	Diagnosis	HV (ml)	HV/kg (ml/kg)	ED (mm)	SF
Total (N = 24)	51.2 (34–69)	CHD 13 CMP 11	1366	18.75	72.3 (N = 22)	0.15 (N = 22)
No pretr. (N = 6) I	51.2 (41–63)	CHD 3 CMP 3	1522	20.5	77.2 (N = 5)	0.12 (N = 5)
ISDN 20 (N = 5) II	53.2 (49–57)	CHD 3 CMP 2	1223	15.7	72.0 (N = 4)	0.21 (N = 4)
ISDN 40 (N = 9) III	49.4 (34–69)	CHD 5 CMP 4	1372	20.0	70.1	0.14
Prazosin (N = 4) IV	51 (47–55)	CHD 2 CMP 2	1348	18.8	70.0	0.13

I   No pretreatment with vasodilators
II   Isosorbide dinitrate 20 mg three times a day
III Isosorbide dinitrate 40 mg three times a day
IV Prazosin 2 mg three times a day

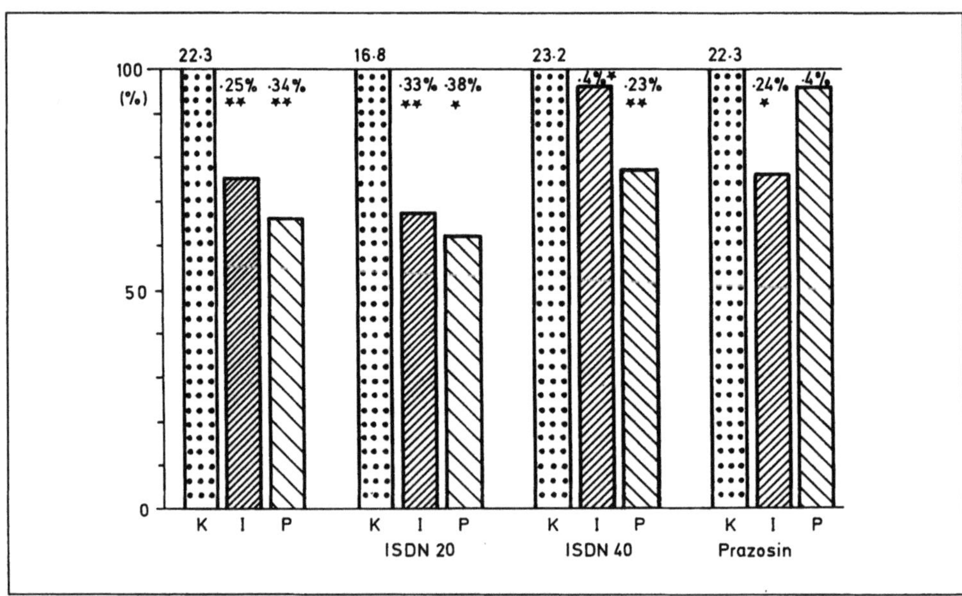

Fig. 4. Acute effect on enddiastolic pulmonary artery pressure (*PAP*) of isosorbide dinitrate (*ISDN*) 40 mg orally in conjunction with ISDN 5 mg sublingually (*I*) or prazosin 2 mg orally (*P*). Previous long-term vasodilator therapy: *No pretr.*, no pretreatment (N = 6); *ISDN 20*, ISDN 20 mg three times a day (N = 5); *ISDN 40*, ISDN 40 mg three times a day (N = 9); *Prazosin*, prazosin 2 mg three times a day (N = 4). *K*, baseline value. *$p < 0.05$; **$p < 0.01$.

82

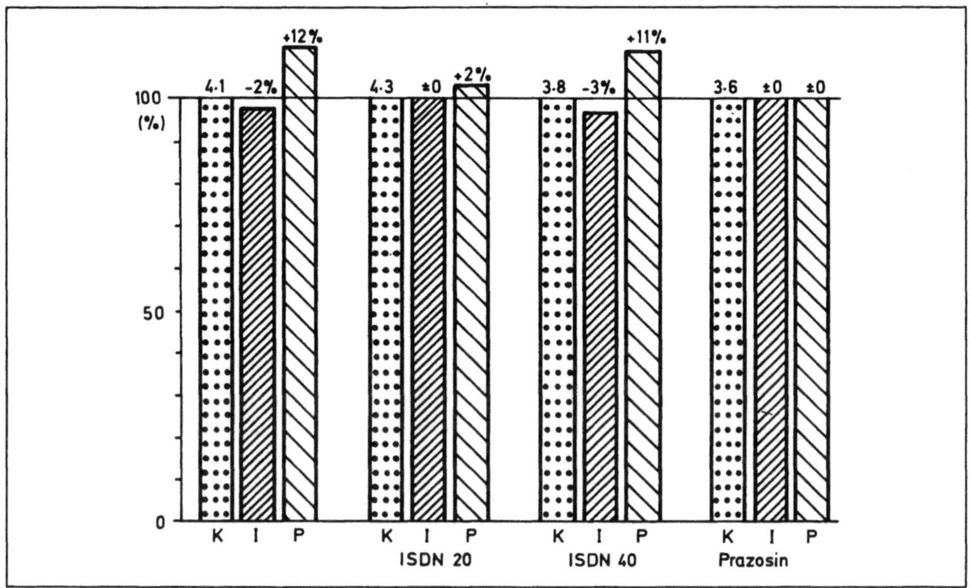

Fig. 5. Acute effect on cardiac output of isosorbide dinitrate (*ISDN*) 40 mg orally in conjunction with ISDN 5 mg sublingually (*I*) or prazosin 2 mg orally (*P*). Previous long-term vasodilator therapy: *No pretr.*, no pretreatment (N = 6); *ISDN 20*, ISDN 20 mg three times a day (N = 5); *ISDN 40*, 40 mg three times a day (N = 9); *Prazosin*, prazosin 2 mg three times a day (N = 4). *K*, baseline values.

As a continuation of this study, our group carried out a further investigation in patients with severe congestive heart failure (N = 24; mean age 51.2 years; heart volume 1366 ml; relative heart volume 18.75 ml/kg; echocardiographic parameters: left-ventricular end-diastolic diameter 72.3 mm, shortening fraction 0.15).

By means of right-heart, flow-directed catheterization, we ascertained the acute effect of ISDN 40 mg orally in conjunction with ISDN 5 mg sublingually or prazosin 2 mg orally in relation to previous long-term vasodilator medication; the sequence of the acutely administered agents was changed systematically. In accordance with the questions posed, we divided the patients into four groups on the basis of the medication they had received for at least 7 days (Table 2):

Group I   (N = 6) no pretreatment with vasodilators
Group II   (N = 5) pretreatment with ISDN 20 mg three times a day
Group III   (N = 9) pretreatment with ISDN 40 mg three times a day
Group IV   (N = 4) pretreatment with prazosin 2 mg three times a day.

Enddiastolic pulmonary artery pressure was elevated to a mean of 22–23 mmHg, with the exception of the group II pretreated with ISDN 20 which had a lower baseline value of 16.8 mmHg (Fig. 4).

In patients not pretreated with vasodilators, the first administration of ISDN or prazosin resulted in a significant reduction in pressure of 25% and 34%, respectively. Patients pretreated with 20 mg ISDN three times a day showed a comparable reaction: a decline in pressure of 33% with ISDN and 38% with prazosin.

By contrast, patients pretreated with 40 mg ISDN three times a day displayed a reduction of only 4% in response to the renewed administration of ISDN, whereas prazosin exerted a reduction of 23%. In patients pretreated with prazosin, a marked decrease in enddiastolic pulmonary artery pressure (–24%) occurred only in response to ISDN; in contrast the renewed administration of prazosin, resulted only in a minimal change of –4%.

Cardiac output (Fig. 5), which displayed mean baseline values between 3.6 l/min (prazosin pretreatment) and 4.3 l/min (ISDN 20 mg pretreatment), was not changed in response to acute ISDN administration in any of the groups. With prazosin, only a slight increase in cardiac output occurred in the group that had not been pretreated (+ 12%) and in the group with ISDN 40 mg pretreatment (+ 11%).

In summary, it can be seen that a thoroughly positive long-term effect can occur during vasodilator therapy. If the individual agents are compared, however, markedly differing effects in terms of long-term therapy appear despite the generally good acute effect. The administration of prazosin in patients with severe myocardial damage appears to have no long-term effect on hemodynamics despite its favorable acute effect. We also noted a comparable pattern of hemodynamic changes using long-term high-dose ISDN therapy.

It should again be mentioned that these two groups of patients showed an immediate hemodynamic response when the drug-type was changed after long-term vasodilator therapy. Reliable acute as well as long-term therapeutic success could be achieved with dihydralazine or relatively low-dose ISDN.

Für die Verfasser:
Prof. Dr. H. Roskamm
Benedikt Kreutz-Rehabilitationszentrum
für Kreislaufkranke
Südring 15
7812 Bad Krozingen

Discussion

ABRAMS:

Did you find a decreased responsiveness of the pulmonary artery diastolic pressure with ISDN as well as with prazosin? Or did ISDN continue to be effective?

HAUF:

After 12 days of ISDN therapy, 20 mg 3 times daily, and after a period of 16 hours without any medication we found a further significant PADP reduction after a new acute dose of ISDN.
With prazosin, control measurement after 12 days of therapy showed no significant reduction of PADP. An additional acute dose of prazosin did not induce any further significant change of the diastolic pulmonary artery pressure.
Almost the same negative response to a new acute dose have been found in the patients who received the high daily dose of 3 times 40 mg ISDN.

ABRAMS:

How can the rather dramatic response to dihydralazine on preload be explained?

HAUF:

We found this effect of the arterial vasodilator in all our patients. Its effect on preload is difficult to explain. It might be a secondary effect.

FRANCIOSA:

We have to be cautious about the importance of hemodynamic changes and we should not extrapolate resting hemodynamics to what can be regarded as a good treatment for chronic heart failure. The data available about therapeutic results are totally contradictary to the hemodynamic data. Prazosin which at rest apparently develops tolerance, is one of the most effective long-term drugs. Hydralazine has striking hemodynamic effects both acutely and chronically, but in the only double-blind trial that I know it had virtually no clinical effects e.g. on exercise capacity as compared to placebo.

HAUF:

These patients were not suitable for exercise testing.

Long-Term Isosorbide Dinitrate Therapy for Pulmonary Hypertension in Patients with Chronic Obstructive Lung Disease

S. Daum, R. Goerg

Introduction

Medical therapy for pulmonary hypertension remains unsatisfactory (4, 6, 16). The majority of drugs exert only a transient effect on pulmonary artery pressure (4, 10, 13, 15). In 1970, Both first reported the favorable effect of isosorbide dinitrate (ISDN) on pulmonary hypertension (1). Subsequent papers confirmed the salutary effect of ISDN on pulmonary artery pressure (4, 8–10, 12, 14). It was generally administered only for a brief period. Both observed no favorable effect in long-term therapy.
Following our use of ISDN in spray or tablet form for short-term investigations (4), we administered ISDN in tablet form for the long-term treatment of patients with chronic obstructive lung disease and precapillary pulmonary hypertension. The work of Eckayam (7) and Lupi-Herrera (12) on primary pulmonary hypertension, published in 1981, was encouraging.

Methods and Patients

In the context of a thorough cardiopulmonary work-up in patients with chronic obstructive lung disease, right-heart catheterization with intracardiac and pulmonary circulation pressure measurements and cardiac output determination by means of thermodilution was carried out; arterial and mixed venous blood gas determination was carried out simultaneously. The investigation was performed at rest (15–20 min), in the "legs up" position, and during exercise (25–50 W).
Once resting steady state values had been reached again following exercise, pressure values, cardiac output, and blood gases were redetermined as baseline levels for ISDN administration. Following the ingestion of one 5-mg tablet sublingually, pressure values in the pulmonary circulation and right atrium were obtained at 5-min intervals. Cardiac output and arterial as well as mixed venous blood gases were determined at 10-min intervals.
Patients then received 20 mg ISDN in sustained-release form three times a day for a period of 6 months. All cardiopulmonary examinations were repeated after 6 months. Values at rest were compared to those obtained during the initial investigation. The patient again received a 5-mg sublingually dose of ISDN check the initial response.
We studied a total of 12 patients (two women and ten men) ranging in age from 32 to 60 years (mean age 48). In two patients treatment had to be discontinued immediately because of arterial hypotension. Ten patients remained for statistical evaluation of the re-

Table 1. Changes in individual parameters for the pulmonary circulation after 6 months of therapy with isosorbide dinitrate (ISDN) 20 mg sustained-release three times a day

	PA$\bar{P}$	$\bar{P}$PCV	CO	PVR	HR	RA$\bar{P}$
N	10	9	9	9	10	10
Declined by						
> 3 mmHg	5		1	2 (< 100 dyn)	1	2
> 6 mmHg	2	7		3 (> 100 dyn)		
Unchanged ± 3 mmHg	3	1	7	2	6	8
Increased	0	1	1	2	3 (> 10 beats/min)	

PA$\bar{P}$, pulmonary artery pressure; $\bar{P}$PCV, pulmonary capillary pressure; CO, cardiac output; PVR, pulmonary vascular resistance; HR, heart rate; RA$\bar{P}$, right atrial pressure

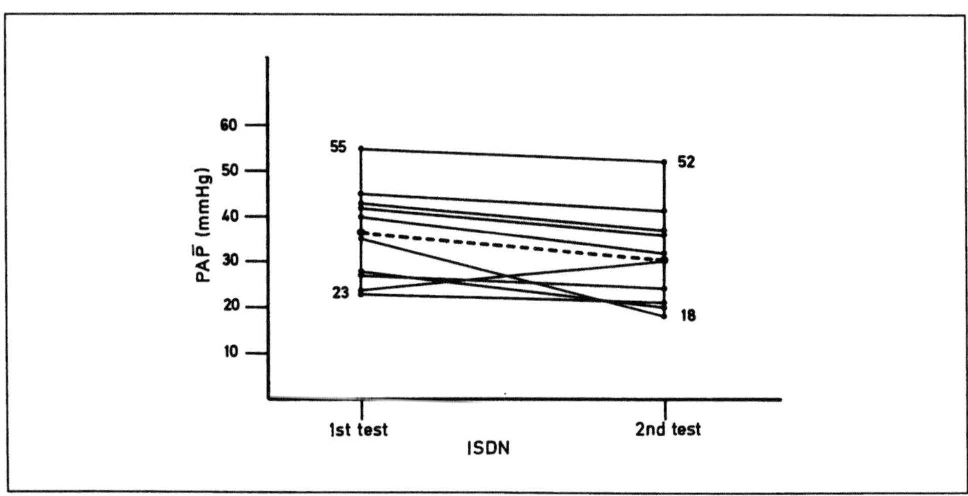

Fig. 1. Mean pulmonary artery pressure (*PA$\bar{P}$*) in individual patients with *chronic obstructive lung disease (N = 10) (solid line)* and mean value (*broken line*) before and after 6 months of therapy with isosorbide dinitrate (*ISDN*) 20 mg sustained-release three times a day. $p < 0.01$.

sults (one woman, nine men). In addition to Isoket*), the patients took Euphyllin tablets or used Sultanol or Berodual aerosol spray. Oxygen therapy and positive-pressure inhalation were not used intentionally.

---

*) Isoket Pharma Schwarz, Euphyllin Byk Gulden , Sultanol Glaxo, Berodual Boehringer Ingelheim

Table 2. Values of mean pulmonary artery pressure (PA$\overline{P}$) and systolic-diastolic pressure (PAB) before and after 20 and 40 mg isosorbide dinitrate respectively

Patient no.	PA$\overline{P}$ (mmHg)		PAB (mmHg)	
	20 mg	40 mg	20 mg	40 mg
1	38	36	120/80	105/70
2	28	24	115/75	105/70
3	32	30	130/80	110/70
4	45	41	125/75	110/70
5	25	26	130/70	100/60

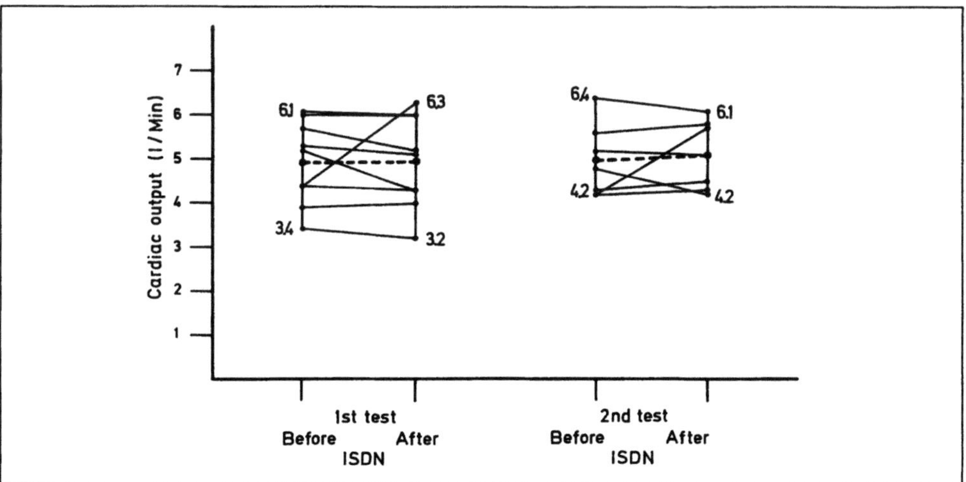

Fig. 2. Cardiac output in individual patients (N = 9) (*solid lines*) in acute tests with 5 mg isosorbide dinitrate (*ISDN*) sublingually before and after 6 months of therapy with ISDN 20 mg sustained-release three times a day. *Broken lines* mean values (changes not significant).

Results

Pulmonary artery pressure is shown in Table 1 and Fig. 1. Mean pressure in the pulmonary artery fell from 36.2 ± 10.6 mmHg to 30.1 ± 10.6 mmHg after 6 months of ISDN therapy. This decline is statistically significant ($p < 0.01$). The reduction in pressure was greater than 6 mmHg in two patientes and between 3 and 5 mmHg in five. In two patients the pressure remained virtually unchanged (± 3 mmHg). A rise was observed in one patient.

Cardiac output (Table 1, Fig. 2) remained virtually unchanged at 6 months in seven patients, fell slightly in one patient, and rose in a single instance.

Pulmonary vascular resistance (Table 1, Fig. 3) showed a decline of more than 100 dyn · s · cm^{-5} in three patients and less than 100 dyn · s · cm^{-5} in two patients. In two further patients it remained unchanged. A rise was observed in two cases.

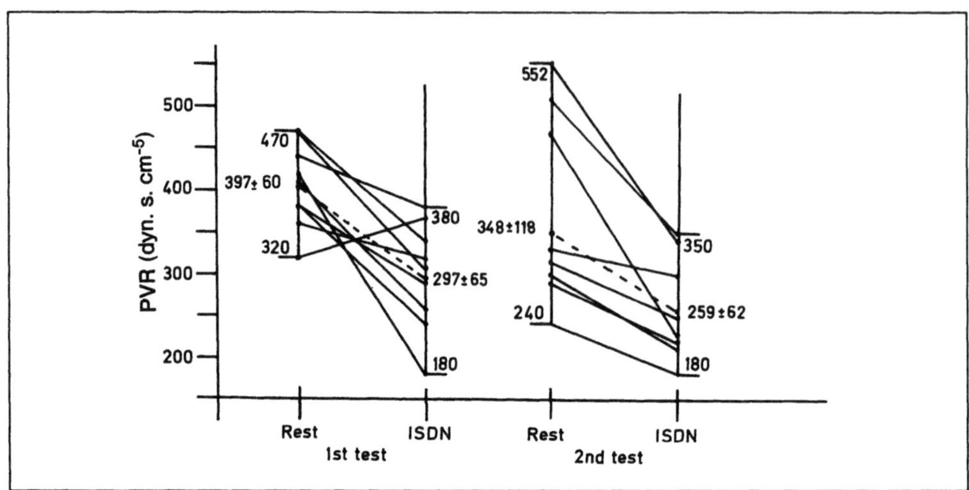

Fig. 3. Pulmonary vascular resistançe (*PVR*) in individual patients (N = 9) (*solid lines*) in acute tests before and after 6 months of acute therapy with isosorbide dinitrate (*ISDN*) 20 mg sustained-release three times a day. *Broken lines*, mean values.

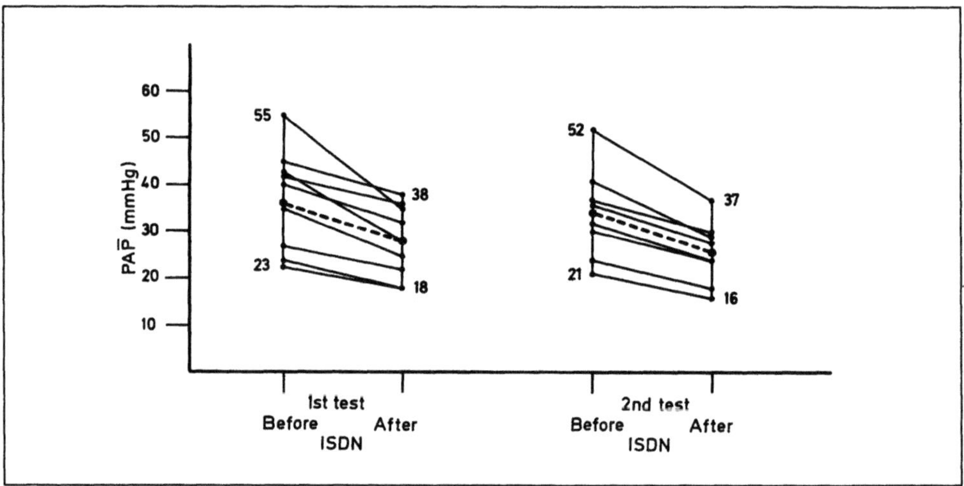

Fig. 4. Mean pulmonary artery pressure (*PA$\overline{P}$)* in individual patients (N = 9) (solid lines) in acute tests with 5 mg isosorbide dinitrate (*ISDN*) sublingually before and after 6 months of therapy with ISDN 20 mg sustained-release three times a day. *Broken lines*, mean values. $p < 0.001$.

Pulmonary artery pressure in acute tests before and after 6 months of ISDN therapy is shown in Fig. 4: the decline after 6 months of ISDN therapy was only moderate. The response of pulmonary artery pressure to the renewed administration of 5 mg ISDN sublingually was as clear in all cases as prior to treatment. Cardiac output had not changed significantly, and pulmonary vascular resistance declined (Fig. 3). This is in agreement with the literature (10, 14) and with the results of our own studies of ISDN inhalation in 1977 (4). The pressure response in the pulmonary artery was maintained even after 6 months

90

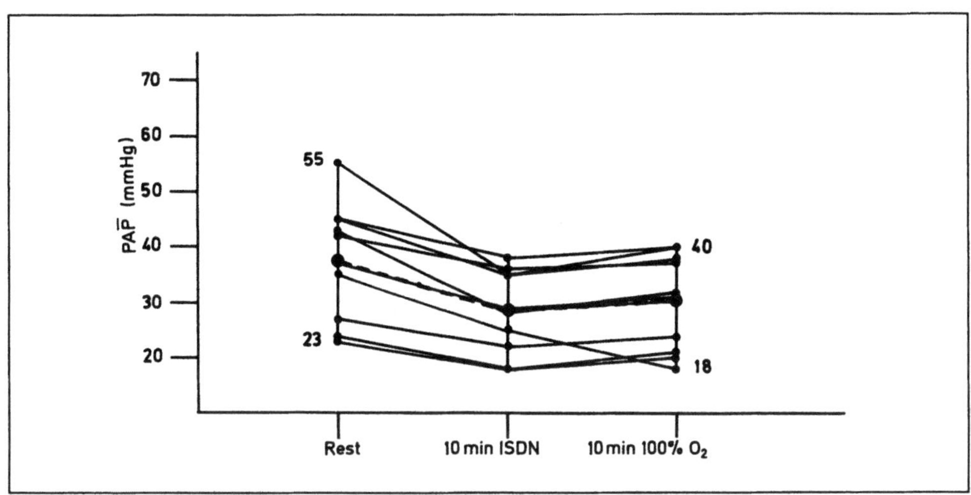

Fig. 5. Mean pulmonary artery pressure *(PAP) in individual patients (N = 9) (solid lines)* at rest as baseline value and 10 min after 5 mg isosorbide dinitrate *(ISDN)* sublingually, in comparison to values after 10 min of 100% oxygen inhalation. In all but one patient, pressure values remained relatively unchanged during oxygen administration. *Broken lines,* mean values, $p < 0.12$.

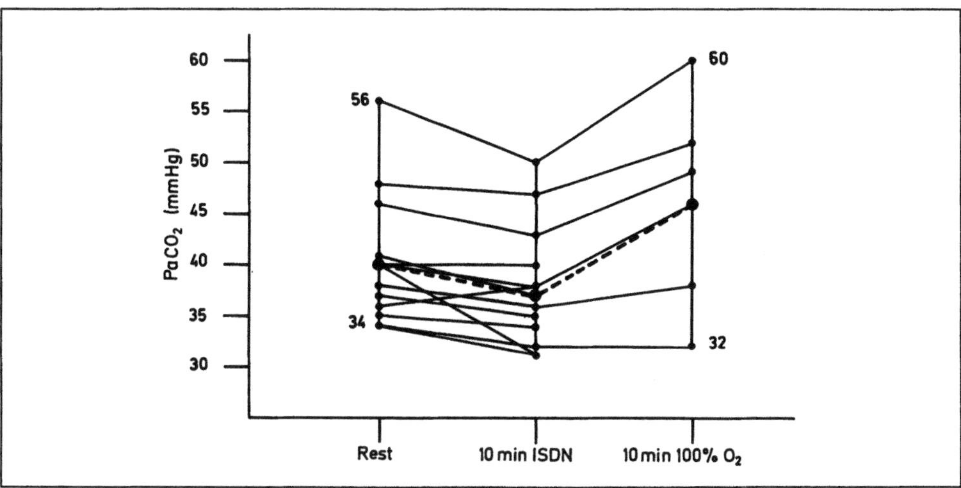

Fig. 6. Arterial carbon dioxide pressure *(PaCO₂)* in individual patients (N = 11) *(solid lines)* at rest during intake of 5 mg isosorbide dinitrate *(ISDN)* sublingually compared to values during 100% oxygen inhalation (N = 6). The pressure rose in four of five patients with chronic obstructive lung disease. This increase is statistically significant compared to the ISDN and initial values. *Broken lines,* mean values, $p < 0.01$.

of therapy and was comparable to the initial test. We could not establish tolerance development.

A comparison of the effect of ISDN with that of 100% oxygen inhalation on mean pulmonary artery pressure (Fig. 5) showed that the decline in mean pressure during oxygen inhalation was not more marked than following ISDN. In only one patient did the pressure in the pulmonary artery decline by more than 8 mmHg. In five cases, on the other

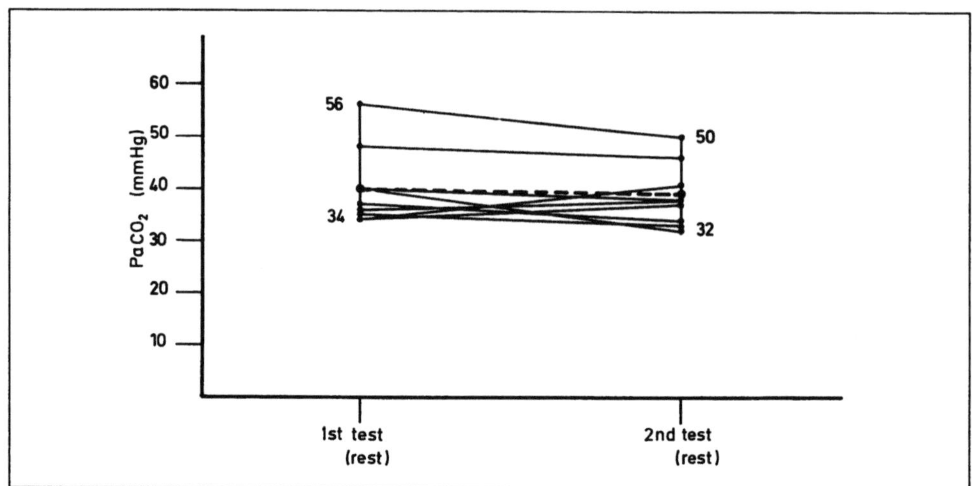

Fig. 7. Arterial carbon dioxide pressure in individual patients (N = 9) (*solid lines*) before and after 6 months of therapy with 20 mg isosorbide dinitrate (*ISDN*) sustained-release three times a day. *Broken line*, mean values (change not significant).

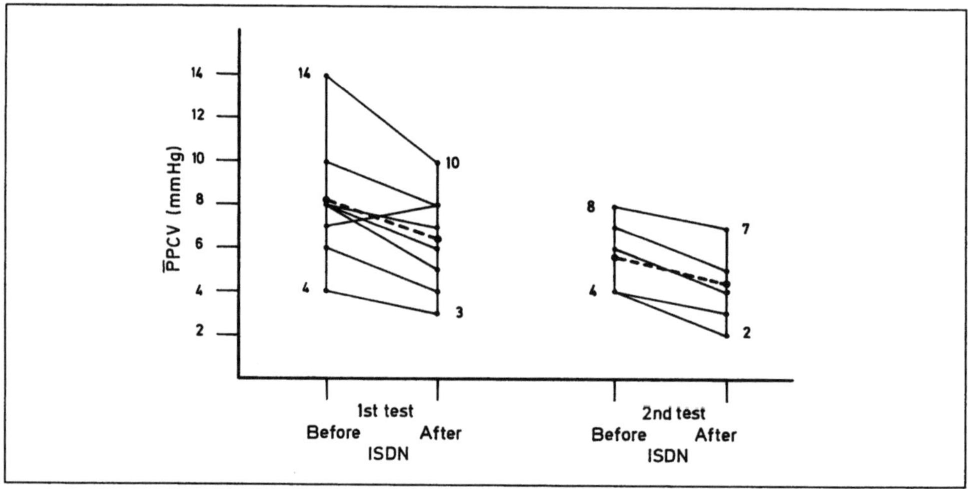

Fig. 8. Mean pulmonary capillary pressure ($\overline{P}PCV$) in individual patients (N = 9) (*solid lines*) during acute tests with 5 mg isosorbide dinitrate (*ISDN*) sublingually before and after 6 months of therapy with 20 mg ISDN sustained-release three times a day. *Broken lines*, mean values (*1st test, p < 0.01; 2nd test, p < 0.05*).

hand, pulmonary artery pressure increased slightly by 2–3 mmHg. This may be related to the increase in arterial carbon dioxide pressure during oxygen inhalation in patients with chronic obstructive lung disease (Fig. 6) in comparison to the initial value. The rise is statistically significant ($p < 0.01$).

During the course of the 6-month treatment period with arterial carbon dioxide pressure remained virtually unchanged (Fig. 7). In three patients it fell by more than 5 mmHg, but we do not view this decline as a result of ISDN therapy.

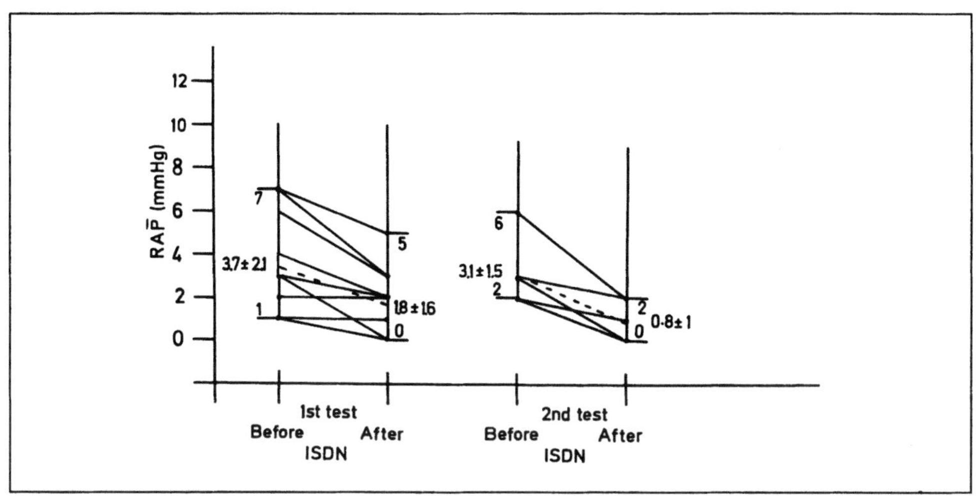

Fig. 9. Mean right atrial pressure *(RAP̄) showed no changes after 6 months of therapy with isosor-*
bide dinitrate (ISDN) 20 mg sustained-release three times a day. In an acute test with 5 mg ISDN
sublingually, RAP̄ fell significantly. *Solid lines,* individual patient values; *broken lines,* mean values.

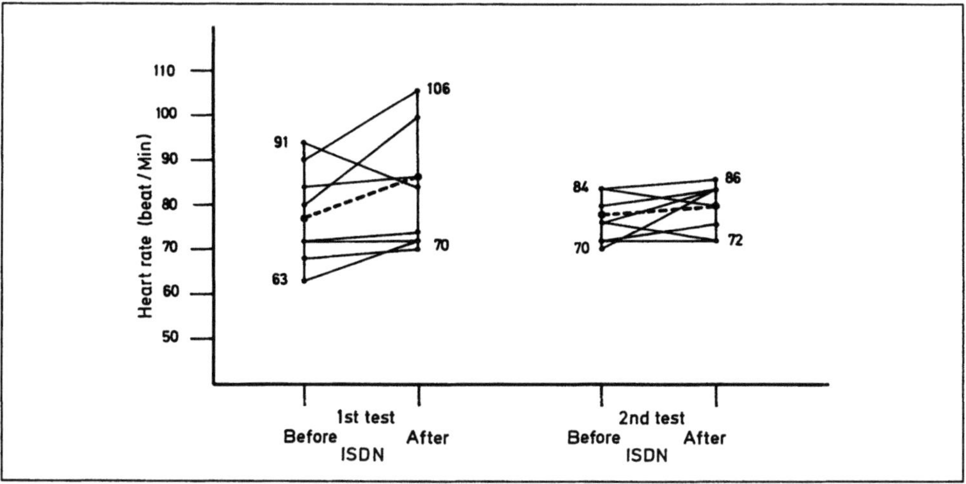

Fig. 10. Heart rate remained virtually unchanged after 6 months of therapy with isosorbide dinitrate
(ISDN) 20 mg sustained-release three times a day. In an acute test with 5 mg ISDN sublingually, before long-term therapy, two patients responded with a rise in heart rate. When the test was repeated
after therapy, the response had stabilized. *Solid lines,* individual patient values (N = 10); *broken
lines,* mean values (changes not significant).

Mean pulmonary capillary pressure was determined in nine patients. In seven of these it
fell by more than 6 mmHg over the 6-month treatment period. It remained unchanged in
one patient (± 3 mmHg) and rose in another. The fall in pressure in the acute tests was
statistically significant, but that following long-term ISDN therapy was not (Fig. 8).
Mean pressure in the right atrium (Table 1, Fig. 9) showed unchanged values after 6
months of ISDN therapy. Mean pressure declined by 3–5 mmHg in two patients and remained unchanged in eight (± 3 mmHg). Here, too, the immediate response to the sub-

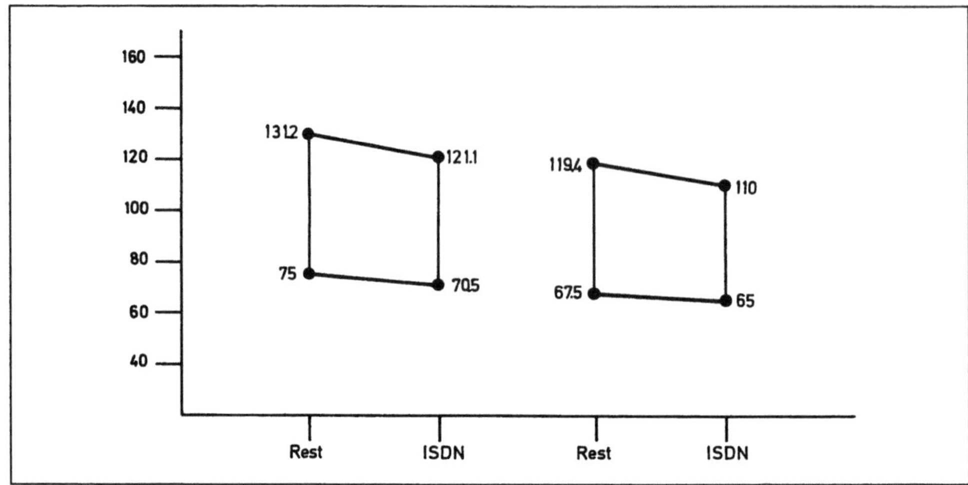

Fig. 11. Systolic and diastolic brachial arterial pressure (mean values in mmHg measured intraarterially) showed a moderate decline over the course of 6 months' therapy with isosorbide dinitrate (*ISDN*) 20 mg sustained-release three times a day. A moderate decrease was also seen during the acute test. $p < 0.005$.

lingual administration of 5 mg ISDN was more favorable than the follow-up value obtained after long-term therapy.

Heart rate (Table 1, Fig. 10) was virtually unchanged at the follow-up examination after 6 months. In the acute tests the heart rate response differed. The low degree of variability in the heart rate response at 6 months following the sublingual administration of 5 mg ISDN was remarkable. Figure 11 shows pressure in the peripheral arteries. Systolic-diastolic arterial pressure at 6 months demonstrated a moderate, insignificant decline in comparison with the initial value.

Discussion

The decline in mean pulmonary artery pressure after 6 months of ISDN therapy constituted an average of 6.1 mmHg. This decline was more pronounced than the fall in mean pulmonary capillary pressure. This confirms our 1977 findings. We assume that the effect of ISDN is exerted not only on the venous side of the pulmonary circulation but predominantly on the arterial side. This is confirmed by the unchanged pressure gradient between pulmonary capillary pressure and diastolic pulmonary artery pressure. Although the decline in pressure during the course of the 6-month treatment period is moderate, the renewed effect of ISDN on the pulmonary circulation represents an additional contribution to the treatment of pulmonary hypertension. This applies not only to precapillary pulmonary hypertension in patients with chronic obstructive lung disease, but also to primary pulmonary hypertension, as our further studies confirmed. The use of ISDN in patients with hypercapnia (hypercapnic acidosis) has advantages over treatment with oxygen inhalation. Pulmonary artery pressure declines, as with oxygen inhalation, but arterial carbon dioxide pressure does not rise, as is the case in some patients with chronic ob-

94

structive lung disease receiving oxygen. We failed to detect a decline in arterial oxygen pressure at follow-up after 6 months of ISDN therapy, as is reported in the literature in short-term studies (2).

Mean right-atrial pressure remained unchanged after 6 months of ISDN therapy. The measurements of acute tests with the sublingual administration of 5 mg ISDN show a pronounced decline in mean right-atrial pressure or enddiastolic right-ventricular pressure (6, 8, 10, 13). Isosorbide dinitrate is presumed not only to affect the region of the pulmonary arteries but also to reduce right-ventricular preload (4, 10, 11).

The renewed administration of ISDN after 6 months of maintenance therapy also causes a decline in mean pulmonary artery pressure and right-atrial pressure (Figs. 4 and 9). This suggests that ISDN administration does not result in tolerance development. The use of 20 mg ISDN in sustained-release form three times a day yielded the same reduction in pulmonary artery pressure as the administration of the identical number of 40-mg tablets. This did not cause an extreme drop in peripheral arterial pressure (Table 2). For these reasons we decided to employ the 20-mg tablets. Two patients were eliminated from the study because of the marked decline in peripheral arterial pressure. These were patients who had had a peripheral systolic arterial pressure of 105 mmHg even prior to therapy. The treatment of precapillary pulmonary hypertension with ISDN enhances the therapeutic possibilities in this condition. It by no means fulfills our preconceptions regarding an effective drug. Isosorbide dinitrate complements existing possibilities especially when patients receiving oxygen inhalation are in danger of hypercapnia in the form of hypercapnic acidosis. The use of ISDN in the treatment of primary pulmonary hypertension is also justified, as the latest studies demonstrate.

Summary

Ten patients with chronic obstructive lung disease and precapillary pulmonary hypertension were treated for 6 months with 20 mg ISDN in sustained-release form three times a day. Follow-up investigations after 6 months showed a decline in mean pulmonary artery pressure of 6 mmHg, whereas the reduction in the pulmonary capillary pressure was only 1.2 mmHg. Cardiac output remained virtually unchanged and pulmonary vascular resistance fell slightly. Follow-up investigations with the acute administration of 5 mg ISDN sublingually showed a uniformly favorable response without any evidence of tolerance development. The effect of ISDN is only partially exerted on the venous side of the pulmonary circulation. The agent acts predominantly on the pulmonary arteries and leads to a reduction in preload on the right heart.

When compared to the effect of 100% oxygen on the pulmonary circulation, the action of ISDN is similar but without the danger of hypercapnia in the form of hypercapnic acidosis, which may occur during oxygen inhalation in patients with chronic obstructive lung disease.

References

1. Both A: Zur Therapie der primären pulmonalen Hypertonie. Z Kreislaufforsch 59: 909 (1970).
2. Chick TW und Mit: The effect of nitroglycerin on gas exchange. A J Med Sc 276: 105 (1978).

3. Daum S, Scheidemandel V, Haselbach G, Goerg R, Chrobok G: Sauerstofftherapie bei chronischem Cor pulmonale. Verhandlungen der Deutschen Gesellschaft für innere Medizin, 81: 499 (1975).

4. Daum S und Mitarbeiter: Isosorbiddinitrat in der Therapie der präkapillären pulmonalen Hypertonie. Atemwegs- und Lungenkrankheiten 4: 538 (1977).

5. Daum S, Goerg R und Schlehe H: ISDN in der Therapie der primären pulmonalen Hypertonie (im Druck).

6. Degenring FH: Die therapeutische Beeinflussung der primär vaskulären Form des chronischen Cor pulmonale und der weiterbestehenden pulmonalen Hypertonie nach Kommissurotomie der Mitralstenose. Z Kreislaufforsch 59: 912 (1970).

7. Elkayam U: Vasodilator therapy in primary pulmonary hypertension. Chest 79: 253 (1981).

8. Geisler LS: Nitrate – Wirkungen auf Herz und Kreislauf. Therapie Woche 3. Int Symp Monte Carlo, Juni 5–7, 1980, S. 11.

9. Härich BKS: Hämodynamik nach Isoket und Isoket Spray beim akuten Herzinfarkt. 1. Nitrat-Symp. Stockholm 1975.

10. Konietzko N, Schlehe H, Härich B, Matthys H: Effect of Isosorbide Dinitrate on Hemodynamics and Respiration of Patients with Coronary Artery Disease and of Patients with Chronic Cor pulmonale. Respiration 32: 368 (1975).

11. Lichtlen PR, Ross RS, Friesinger GC, Beruster L: Die Wirkung von Nitroglyzerin auf die Koronardurchblutung unter Berücksichtigung der selektiven Koronarographie und Messung der Koronardurchblutung mit Xenon 133. Cardiologia 48: 371 (1966).

12. Lupi-Herrera E, Bialostozky D, and Sobrino A: The Role of Isoproterenol in Pulmonary Artery Hypertension of Unknown Etiology (Primary). Chest 79: 292 (1981).

13. Olesch KG, Belz G, Heesemann E: Einfluß von Isosorbitdinitrat auf den Pulmonalarteriendruck beim chronischen Cor pulmonale. Arzneim Forsch (Drug Res) 11: 1876 (1972).

14. Pantzer M: Wirkung von Isosorbiddinitrat auf den Pulmonalarteriendruck. Med Welt 29: 1494 (1978).

15. Renggli I und Daum S: Obstruktive pulmonale Hypertension: Wirkung von Aminophyllin, Hyperventilation und O_2-Atmung. Schweiz med Wschr 101: 352 (1971).

16. Wood P: Diseases of the heart and circulation. Egre & Spotliswode, London 1956.

Authors' address:
Prof. Dr. S. Daum
Pulmonologische Abteilung der
I. Med. Klinik der TU
Ismaninger Str. 22
8000 München 80

Discussion

KOBER:

Are your patients comparable to patients with coronary heart disease in respect to their pressures under resting conditions?

GOERG:

Our patients had pulmonary hypertension because of their chronic obstructive lung disease, but there was no left or right heart failure. The pressures were normal.

FOX:

Can you tell us about the treatment of pulmonary hypertension with nitrates?

GOERG:

There was a fall of the mean pulmonary artery pressure of 6 mm between the beginning of the therapy and after 6 months. Only when giving an additional 5 mg of Isoket, we had a higher fall of 9 mm of mercury. What we wanted to do is to show that we can use ISDN in pulmonary hypertension, because there is little chance to treat this disease, or this complication of chronic lung disease, and there is one big advantage compared to continuously giving pure oxygen because in chronic obstructive lung disease there is always the danger of the rising carbon dioxide level in the blood during continuous oxygen breathing.

FOX:

Can these results be compared with the effects that are being seen with calcium antagonists?

GOERG:

I should assume it, but we don't have any experience of our own.

FRANCIOSA:

You showed us haemodynamic improvement. What happened with regard to symptoms, exercise tolerance, blood gases, ventilation function etc.?

GOERG:

There was no improvement of partial oxygen pressure in the arterial blood. If a patient has a mean pressure of about 35 mm mercury in the pulmonary artery, this is a very severe obstructive lung disease. We are satisfied to avoid a further rise in pulmonary arterial pressure.

FRANCIOSA:

That is also our experience. We studied a similar group of patients a couple of years ago and more or less abandoned the idea of unloading the right ventricle, because we could only show small pressure changes at this magnitude, but there was really no change at all in the patients' clinical status, pulmonary function and exercise tolerance.

GOERG:

Probably there is no change in oxygen uptake and maximal oxygen uptake, but the patients feel better. Dyspnoea may be correlated to pulmonary hypertension rather than to ventilation disturbances. But it is difficult to quantify dyspnoea.

DANAHY:

Let me back up Dr. Franciosa's comments. We studied a group of patients with COPD and significant pulmonary hypertension, and similarly found that you can lower pulmonary artery pressure, but not to a marked degree. Are you routinely putting patients with pulmonary hypertension on ISDN, and if so, what doses are you using?

GOERG:

We had some patients in the beginning who had 40 mg 3 times a day, the double dose. And the effects were not better than with 20 mg 3 times a day.
We use ISDN in pulmonary hypertension because we have nothing else except oxygen.

KOBER:

What do you think is the mechanism of action? We have studied pulmonary circulation by angiography and have seen in coronary patients that there are increases in venous diameters, but no, or only very slight, increases in the diameters of the small pulmonary arteries. In your patients you found no change in cardiac output. Do you think that in chronic pulmonary hypertension due to lung disease there is a possibility to dilate the pulmonary arteries, or is there an opening of arteriovenous shunts?

GOERG:

I do not think there was shunt opening, because in this case the partial oxygen pressure would have fallen; but this was not the case. Perhaps the difference between diastolic pulmonary artery pressure and mean pulmonary capillary pressure decreases, therefore I said we did not observe a change in pulmonary vascular resistance, but perhaps this is wrong statistically. There could have been a drop in pulmonary vascular resistance.

Development of Tolerance and Peripheral Hemodynamic Effects of Molsidomine

H. Kaiser, G. Sold, J. Schrader, and H. Kreuzer

With increasing use of vasoactive substances in the treatment of patients with coronary artery disease, with and without angina pectoris, with and without congestive heart failure, one must consider the possibility that, as a result of different mechanisms, tolerance to the desired hemodynamic effects of these substances may occur. Indeed, in the case of nitrates there is increasing evidence that tolerance at least to some of these effects may develop (1): for example, isosorbide dinitrate given chronically leads to significantly lesser changes in heart rate, blood pressure, and exercise-induced ST deviations than occur with a single dose (2). However, the clinical significance of tolerance to singular effects is unclear; at present there are no convincing reports that tolerance extends to patients with congestive heart failure and to antianginal effects (3).

With molsidomine, a recent alternative to the nitrate group of drugs (4), the possibility again arises that tolerance to desired or undesired therapeutic effects may occur. This study was designed to define the peripheral hemodynamic effects of molsidomine in relation to nitroglycerin, and to compare single-dose effects of molsidomine with changes obtained after several days' treatment in order to evaluate short-term tolerance.

Heart rate and systolic and diastolic blood pressure were measured in 12 healthy volunteers, in a supine position and after 5 min standing (Fig. 1), and again while supine and while standing following sublingual administration of 1.6 mg nitroglycerin. In addition,

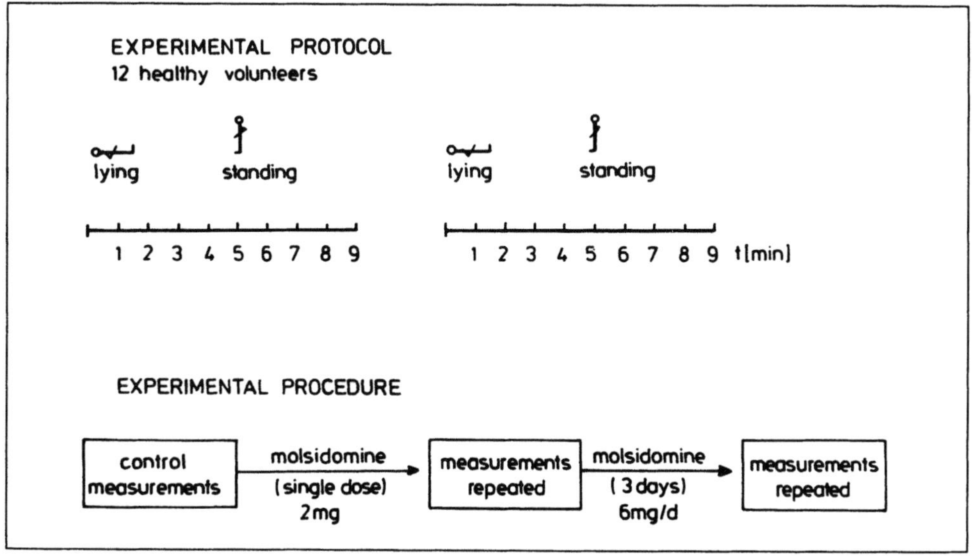

Fig. 1. a Experimental protocol (N = 12); **b** experimental procedure.

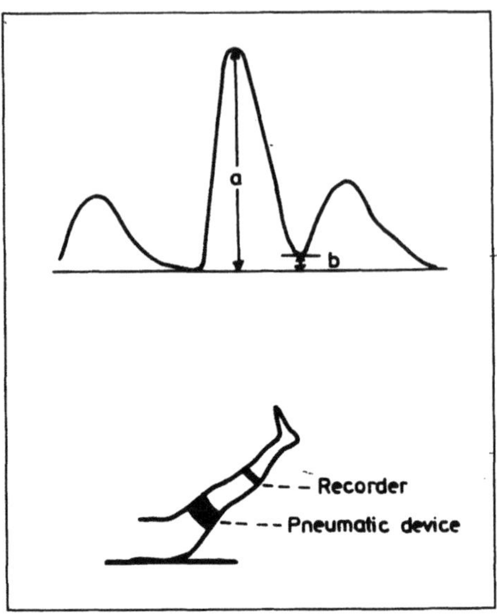

Fig. 2. a Ratio (a : b) between systolic maximal and diastolic minimal flow determined by acral oscillometry; b venous volume of the calf (ml/100 ml tissue).

acral oscillometry was performed after 4 min supine and after 4 min standing, both before and after nitroglycerin; peripheral arterial vasodilatation was estimated by the ratio a : b (Fig. 2) between systolic maximal and diastolic minimal flow (5). During each supine period, venous volume of the calf was measured by the occlusion technique using the strain gauge plethysmograph (6).

When the control measurements had been taken, molsidomine (2 mg) was given orally; the measurements were repeated after 90 min. Molsidomine was continued on a 6-mg/day regimen; the measurements were repeated 3 days later and again 90 min after the last single dose. From individual data the arithmetic mean ($\pm$ SEM) was computed; differences observed were compared by using Student's t-test for paired data.

As expected (Fig. 3), heart rate increased and systolic blood pressure decreased significantly when the subject was standing rather than lying, and there were only insignificant changes in diastolic blood pressure and a : b ratio. With nitroglycerin heart rate increased further, systolic blood pressure decreased, and a : b ratio increased, more so in the supine than in the standing position ($p < 0.05$).

Comparing data obtained after 3 min in the supine and after 3 min in the standing position, heart rate was 76.5 $\pm$ 3.4 beats/min and 93.3 $\pm$ 3.75 beats/min respectively, and after nitroglycerin 80.9 $\pm$ 3.32 beats/min and 104.2 $\pm$ 4.36 beats/min respectively (Fig. 4). Heart rate after molsidomine (single dose) was 72.4 $\pm$ 3.03 beats/min in the supine position, 100.6 $\pm$ 6.08 beats/min while standing ($p < 0.05$); 3 min following nitroglycerin administration it was 82.4 $\pm$ 3.12 beats/min and 107.1 $\pm$ 7.43 beats/min respectively ($p < 0.05$). Three days later, heart rate was 73.4 $\pm$ 2.69 beats/min and 94.5 $\pm$ 5.34 beats/min before, and 80.1 $\pm$ 5.16 beats/min and 100.7 $\pm$ 4.35 beats/min after nitroglycerin ($p < 0,05$).

Control measurements for systolic blood pressure were 117.1 $\pm$ 3.67 mmHg while supine, 107.1 $\pm$ 2.57 mmHg while standing, decreasing with nitroglycerin to 113.8 $\pm$ 2.68 mmHg and 102.9 $\pm$ 2.77 mmHg respectively ($p < 0.05$). After molsidomine (single dose),

102

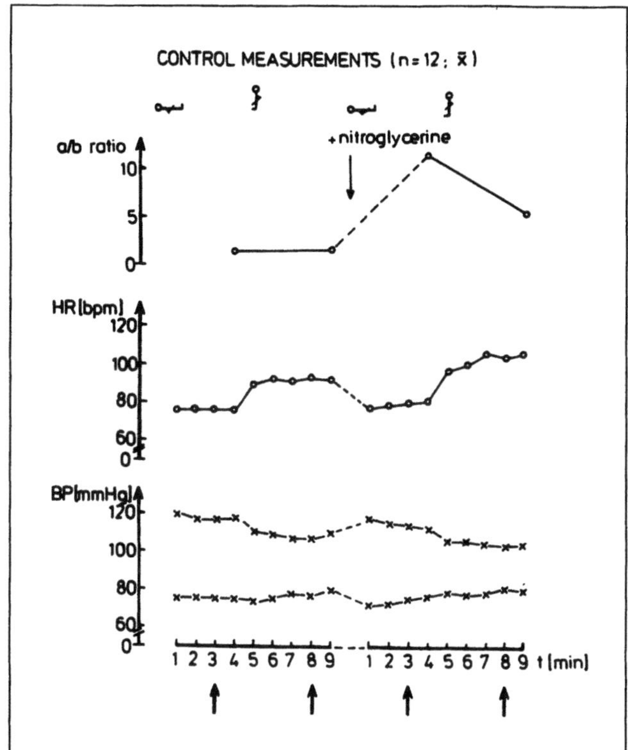

Fig. 3. Control measurements (N = 12, X).

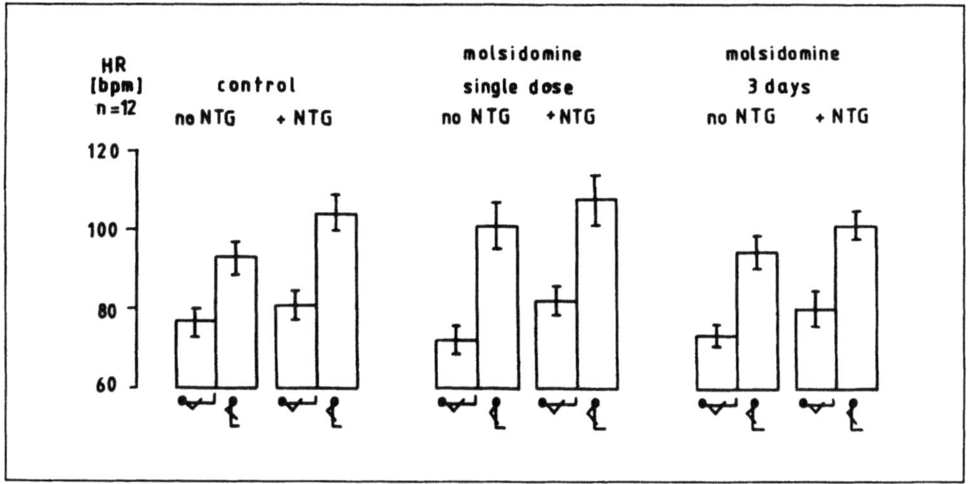

Fig. 4. Effects of nitroglycerin (*NTG*) on heart rate (*HR*) measured at control, after single-dose molsidomine, and after 3 days of molsidomine (N = 12).

systolic blood pressure was 108.8 ± 2.64 mmHg while supine, 101.9 ± 1.87 while standing; after nitroglycerin it was 102.5 ± 2.32 mmHg and 94.4 ± 2.58 mmHg (all differences significant).

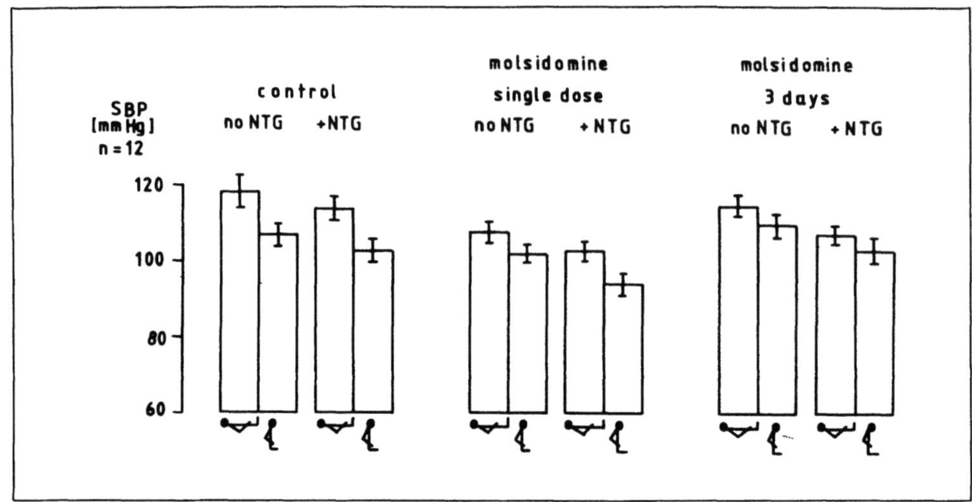

Fig. 5. Effects of nitroglycerin (*NTG*) on systolic blood pressure (*SBP*) measured at control, after single-dose molsidomine, and after 3 days of molsidomine (N = 12).

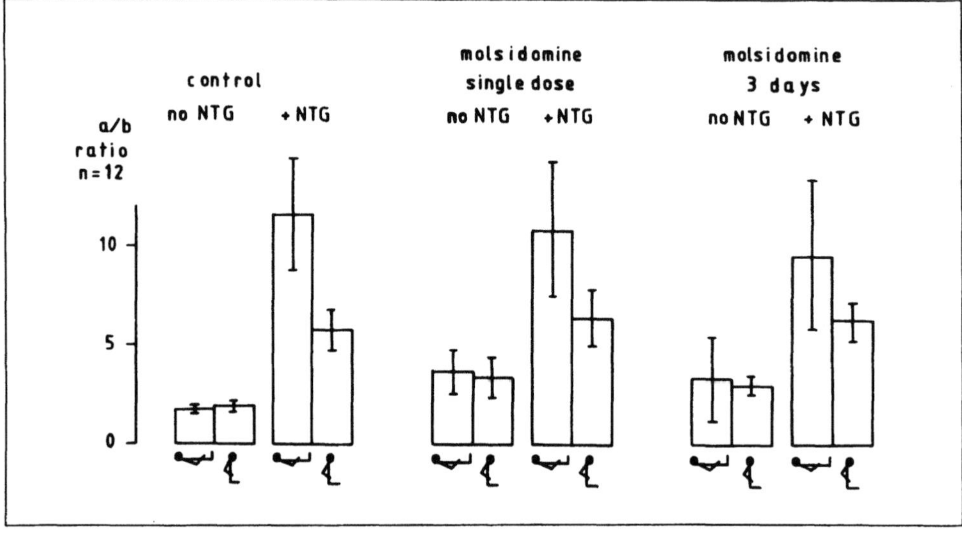

Fig. 6. Effects of nitroglycerin (*NTG*) on ratio between systolic maximal and diastolic minimal flow (*a : b ratio*) measured at control, after single-dose molsidomine, and after 3 days of molsidomine (N = 12).

Three days later, systolic blood pressure (Fig. 5) was 115 ± 2.05 mmHg while supine and 109.8 ± 2.8 mmHg while standing before nitroglycerin, and 108.1 ± 2.14 mmHg and 103.7 ± 2.63 mmHg after nitroglycerin (all $p<0.05$). When absolute values for heart rate and systolic blood pressure were compared, no difference was found between control, single-dose molsidomine, and 3 days of molsidomine ($p<0.05$).

104

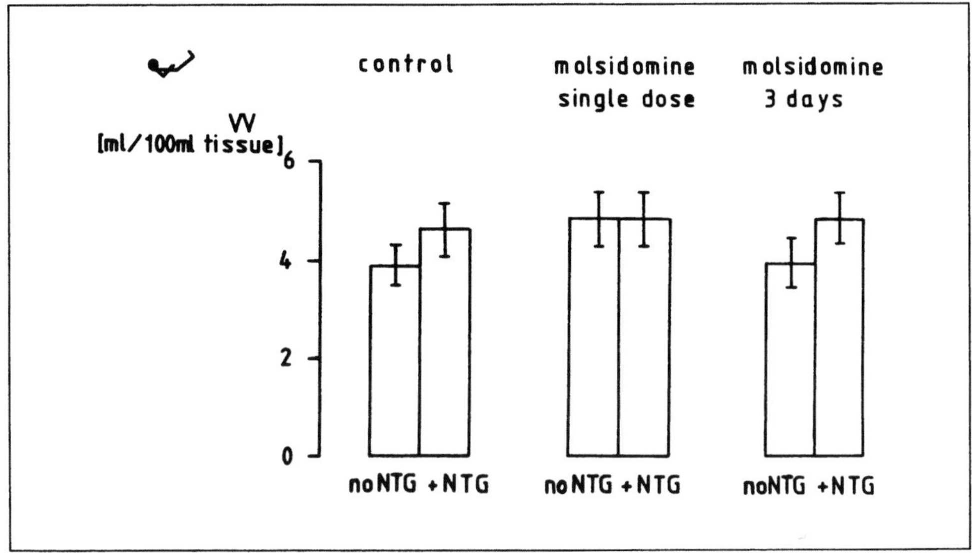

Fig. 7. Effects of nitroglycerin (*NTG*) on venous volume of the calf (*VV*) measured control after single-dose molsidomine, and after 3 days of molsidomine (N = 12).

Control a : b ratio (Fig. 6) was 1.7 $\pm$ 0.09 while supine, 1.8 $\pm$ 0.14 while standing; after nitroglycerin it increased significantly to 11.6 $\pm$ 2.77 and 5.7 $\pm$ 0.98 respectively. After single-dose molsidomine, a : b ratio was 3.51 $\pm$ 0.92 and 3.34 $\pm$ 0.86 (NS) before, 10.96 $\pm$ 3.39 and 6.4 $\pm$ 1.23 after nitroglycerin (all $p < 0.05$). Three days later the corresponding values were 3.4 $\pm$ 1.3 and 3 $\pm$ 0.52 before, and 9.7 $\pm$ 2.66 and 6.3 $\pm$ 1.21 after nitroglycerin. Thus, while both molsidomine and nitroglycerin increased the a : b ratio ($p < 0.05$), the latter proved to be more effective, and the result was even better when both drugs were given simultaneously ($p < 0.05$).

Venous volume of the calf expressed as ml/100 ml tissue was 3.9 $\pm$ 0.39, and increased to 4.7 $\pm$ 0.52 after nitroglycerin ($p < 0.05$). Under molsidomine venous capacity increased to 4.8 $\pm$ 0.54 ml/100 ml (single dose), with no additional effect of nitroglycerin (Fig. 7). However, under comparable conditions 3 days later venous volume had returned to 3.93 $\pm$ 0.47 ml/100 ml; the addition of nitroglycerin led to an increase to 4.83 $\pm$ 0.5 ml/100 ml.

Regarding heart rate and systolic blood pressure, the data obtained confirm reports stating that molsidomine influences both parameters less than does nitroglycerin (Fig. 6). Acral oscillometry, however, shows that molsidomine leads to peripheral arterial dilatation with a : b ratio increasing by 76% – 106%. In this respect there is no difference between single dose and 3-day regimen, both being surpassed by nitroglycerin.

As for venous capacity, single-dose molsidomine leads to an increase of 24%, comparable to the effect of nitroglycerin. When both drugs are taken simultaneously no further increase is seen. Venous volume measured after molsidomine has been taken for 3 days returns to normal, however, an effect reversed 3 min after application of nitroglycerin.

Thus, when the various hemodynamic parameters are compared, molsidomine differs from nitroglycerin with regard to heart rate, systolic blood pressure, and the amount of peripheral arterial dilatation; although there is a comparable increase in venous volume with both drugs, this effect is lost with molsidomine taken for 3 days, indicating that for venous capacity tolerance may develop.

References

1. Schrey A: Toleranz bei Nitropräparaten? Medizinische Klinik 76: 699 (1981).
2. Markis JE, Gorlin R, Mills RM, Williams RA, Schweitzer P, Ransil BJ: Amer J Cardiol 43: 265 (1979).
3. Danahy, DT, Burwell DT, Aronow WS, Prakash R: Sustained hemodynamic and antianginal effect of high dose oral isosorbide dinitrate. Circulation 55: 381 (1977).
4. Lochner W, Grund E, Müller-Ruchholtz E-R, Lapp ER: Vergleichende Untersuchungen über die Wirkung von Molsidomin und Nitroglyzerin auf das kapazitiv-venöse System des großen Kreislaufs. 1. Molsidomin-Symposion, München 1978, Ed. W. Lochner, Urban und Schwarzenberg, München-Wien-Baltimore, 1979.
5. Schlup P, Zatti Ch, Studer H: Toleranzentwicklung gegenüber den haemodynamischen Wirkungen von Nitroglyzerin. Schweiz Med Wochenschr 110: 1927 (1980).
6. Becker HM, Klemm J: Zur Wertigkeit der Dehnungsmeßstreifen-Stauplethysmographie. Herz/Kreisl. 4: 254 (1972).

Author's address:
Dr. H. Kaiser
Medizinische Klinik und Poliklinik
der Universität Göttingen
Robert-Koch-Str. 40
3400 Göttingen

Discussion

KOBER:

Dr. Kaiser, do you think that the tolerance to the effect on venous volume is the same for nitroglycerin and for molsidomine regardless whether you treat the patient first with molsidomine or nitroglycerin?

KAISER:

No, I think that the tolerance development is seen for molsidomine only in this study, because when a single dose of molsidomine is given first and nitroglycerin afterwards, there is no increase of venous volume at this moment. Three days later, there is a significant decrease of venous volume compared to the acute dose. And when nitroglycerin is administered at that time, there is the same increase as in the control test. So I think this is an effect of molsidomine rather than a problem of nitroglycerin. We did not study the long-term effect of nitroglycerin on venous volume and the additional effect of molsidomine.

BACHMANN:

You measured the venous volume in the periphery by plethysmography. Is this representative of the whole system?

KAISER:

I am sure it is not representative of the whole system. The intra-abdominal veins are very important for the increase of venous capacity. With plethysmography we only measure the venous volume of the calf.

BECKER:

Dr. Kaiser, your data suggest that tolerance cannot occur at the receptor site. I can not belive that the molsidomine receptor is the same as the nitrate receptor. Do you agree?

KAISER:

I can not comment on this.

BUSSMANN:

At what time after last dose of molsidomine did you measure, and which were the highest molsidomine doses? Did higher molsidomine doses have more pronounced effects?

KAISER:

We measured 90 minutes after the last dose of molsidomine. The dose was 6 mg/day. We didn't use higher doses.

KOBER:

Just a brief comment:
By echocardiogram we studied the capacity and volume of the abdominal veins and found an increase in venous volume after nitroglycerin. Thus the increase of venous volume seems to be a common change throughout the body and the change in the calf veins is possibly representative for the whole system. But there may be differences in the amount of change because there is a difference in the anatomy of the veins. The veins in the calves have more developed vascular musculature than the veins in the abdomen or in the lungs.

Acute and Chronic Effects of Oral Isosorbide Dinitrate in Patients with Angina

D. T. Danahy

Nineteen men with chronic, stable effort angina were studied. All patients had a history of clearly documented myocardial infarction and/or coronary angiographic demonstration of greater than 70% luminal narrowing in at least one major coronary artery. No patient had hypertension or congestive heart failure at entry into the study.

Propranolol was tapered and stopped 72 h prior to study. No patient received digoxin or diuretics during the study.

Patients were hospitalized for 5 days during both the initial testing and the follow-up testing. Patients were exercised on a graded protocol using a constant-load bicycle ergometer to the onset of angina. At least two practice exercise tests were performed prior to definitive testing. Simultaneous ECG monitoring of leads II and V5 was performed throughout the test, including the first 6 min following exercise. Heart rates were measured from the ECG recordings. Blood pressure was measured using a mercury sphygmomanometer. Heart rate and blood pressure were both measured in a sitting position.

The isosorbide dinitrate (ISDN) dose was selected on an individual basis by monitoring heart rate and blood pressure response after ISDN. An attempt was made to maximize ISDN dosage while avoiding severe headaches or a precipitous fall in blood pressure. All patients had at least a 10-mmHg fall in systolic blood pressure and/or a 10-beat/min increase in heart rate after the chosen ISDN dose. The mean dose of ISDN was 29 mg.

On the 3rd day in hospital patients were exercised twice with 2 h between the tests. Patients were given 0.4 mg nitroglycerin or a placebo sublingually in a randomized double-blind crossover fashion 2 min prior to exercise.

On the 4th and 5th days in hospital, patients were given a control exercise test followed after 15 min by oral drug administration. Exercise tests were then performed at 1, 3 and 5 h after drug administration. Patients were given ISDN and a placebo of identical appearance orally in a randomized double-blind crossover manner.

After the initial study patients continued taking their individual dose of ISDN four times a day. Patients then returned after a mean of 5.6 months for follow-up testing using the same protocol. Isosorbide dinitrate was stopped 14 h before follow-up testing.

Initial testing showed a 56% (p < 0.001) longer exercise time after sublingual nitroglycerin than after sublingual placebo. At follow-up testing, the exercise time was 51% longer after sublingual nitroglycerin (p < 0.001) than after placebo. There was no significant difference between initial testing and follow-up testing as regards the exercise times following sublingual nitroglycerin.

The mean heart rate increase measured 2 min after sublingual nitroglycerin, immediately prior to exercise, was 9.9 beats/min (p < 0.001) at initial testing. At follow-up testing, the mean heart rate increase 2 min after sublingual nitroglycerin was 8.3 beats/min (p < 0.001). The mean fall in systolic blood pressure measured 2 min following sublingual nitroglycerin was 11.3 mmHg (p < 0.001) at initial testing and 7.1 mmHg (p < 0.002) at follow-up testing. There was no significant difference between initial testing and follow-up testing as regards systolic blood pressure and heart rate changes after sublingual nitroglycerin.

Initial testing at 1 h after oral drug administration showed a 58% (p < 0.05) longer mean exercise time following ISDN than following placebo. At follow-up testing, there was also a 58% (p < 0.005) better result after ISDN than after placebo. At 3 h after ISDN, mean exercise time was improved by 38% (p < 0.05) initially and by 27% (p < 0.005) on follow-up testing. At 5 h after ISDN, mean exercise time was improved by 13% (NS) initially and by 21% (p < 0.02) at follow-up testing. There are no significant differences between initial and follow-up exercise times after ISDN.

The response to oral ISDN paralleled the response to sublingual nitroglycerin. The patients who demonstrated the best response to sublingual nitroglycerin generally showed a good response to oral ISDN. Patients showing less improvement after sublingual nitroglycerin also showed less benefit from oral ISDN.

Resting heart rate was significantly increased between 15 min and 5 h after ISDN at initial testing. The peak increase in heart rate was 18 beats/min (p < 0.001) at 1 h after ISDN. Resting heart rate was also significantly increased between 15 min and 5 h after ISDN at follow-up testing. However, the heart rate changes at follow-up testing were consistently less than those seen at initial testing. At 1 h after ISDN during follow-up testing, the mean heart rate was increased by 12 beats/min more than in placebo cases (p < 0.01). This was significantly less than the 18-beat/min difference seen at initial testing (p < 0.05). The mean heart rate increase over the entire 5-h study was 10.2 beats/min initially and 6.1 beats/min at follow-up testing. This difference of 4.1 beats/min is significant (p < 0.001).

Resting systolic blood pressure was decreased between 15 min and 5 h after ISDN during initial testing. The peak fall in systolic blood pressure was 19 mmHg (p < 0.001) at 1 h after ISDN. Resting systolic blood pressure was also decreased between 15 min and 5 h after ISDN at follow-up. However, at follow-up testing the systolic blood pressure changes were consistently less than the changes seen with initial testing. At 1 h after ISDN during follow-up testing, systolic blood pressure was decreased by 14 mmHg (p < 0.001) more than in placebo cases. This was less than the 19-mmHg discrepancy seen at initial testing, but the 5-mmHg difference is not significant. The mean decrease in systolic blood pressure over the entire 5-h study was 11.6 mmHg initially and 8.7 mmHg at follow-up testing. This difference of 2.9 mmHg is significant (p < 0.001).

These data show significant improvement in exercise time to angina at 1 and 3 h after oral ISDN during acute testing. This improvement was maintained during follow-up testing after 5.6 months of therapy with oral ISDN. Similarly, exercise time to angina was improved after sublingual nitroglycerin in these same patients during acute testing. Follow-up testing with sublingual nitroglycerin after 5.6 months of oral ISDN therapy showed the effect of sublingual nitroglycerin to be maintained.

A fall in resting systolic blood pressure and an increase in resting heart rate were noted after sublingual nitroglycerin and between 15 min and 5 h after oral ISDN on initial testing. At follow-up testing these changes persisted, but the effect was attenuated.

In conclusion, these data show partial hemodynamic tolerance to the effect of oral ISDN in angina patients after chronic use. However, there was no demonstrable tolerance in the antianginal efficacy of oral ISDN with chronic use, nor was there any demonstrable cross-tolerance to the antianginal effect of sublingual nitroglycerin.

112

Author's address:
Dr. D. T. Danahy
37 Oxwood Circle
Madison, Wisconsin 53717

Discussion

FOX:

The fall in systolic blood pressure after 5 months of therapy was less pronounced, and interpreted as partial tolerance. What were the initial systolic pressure values?

DANAHY:

The control values were about the same, but fell to a lesser degree after 5 months.

FOX:

What were your criteria for exercise time and what was the rate-pressure-product? Was there any difference between the pre- and post-5-months-period?

DANAHY:

The patients were exercised on a bicycle ergometer. We individualized the tests which were done initially and after 5 months. The exercise times were between 3 and 6 minutes.
Exercise was stopped after onset of angina pectoris. In the majority of patients there were significant ST-changes at the point the test was stopped because of angina.

FOX:

Was there any difference if you looked at the ST-segment changes at the beginning of angina. It is difficult for the patients to remember how severe angina was 5 months ago.

DANAHY:

Generally we found that with nitrates the exercise times were prolonged, but the degree of ST-segment change at the time they stopped were the same with control versus drug. They also were not different from initial to follow-up testing. There was one patient who was no longer experiencing angina as a consistent end-point for the test; so the follow-up testing and his data were actually excluded from analysis for that reason. On several of the follow-up tests this patient exercised to the point of exhaustion without developing angina, even when he was receiving placebo on control tests.

BACHMANN:

There are some differences between the action of nitrates on the venous and on the arterial system. Since you found no decrease in blood pressure during follow-up exercise testing and there were not statistically significant changes between initial testing and follow-up testing, does that point to tolerance prevailing in the arterial system?

DANAHY:

I am not certain that the fall in systolic pressure is merely a reflection of the arterial effects of the nitrates, it may be primarily a venous effect with a decreased venous return. With our protocol we can't separate those effects. The difference between systolic blood pressure fall, initially and during follow-up, is not significant looking on any given point of the curve, but there were consistent changes throughout the 5-months-period. The mean of all those blood pressure values shows a highly significant change from initial to follow-up testing. I believe this to be some evidence of tolerance to the vasodilating effects of the drug.

KALTENBACH:

You mentioned a mean single dose of 29 mg ISDN. Would you today still consider this to be a very high dose?

DANAHY:

Today much higher doses of nitrates are used. At the time we initiated the study the dose we used was considered a very large one. In some of the earlier studies 5 mg or 10 mg have been used. There is still a problem if one starts with large doses, because of the headaches. So for starting doses I still think 29 mg are a substantial mean dose. I have to admit, however, that our concept has considerably changed during these last years.

KENEDI:

If I understood correctly, you didn't find any difference after 5 months in the degree of ST-segment depression following isosorbide dinitrate.
One should not speak about nitrate tolerance if you did not find any differences in this relevant parameter.

DANAHY:

We also found no difference in the exercise times from control to 5 months. Our end-point was angina. In many patients the ST-segment change at the onset of angina was the same, although with nitrates the patients were able to exercise for a longer period before they reached that end-point. We regard this end-point as better than an arbitrarily selected time.
I can't answer your question about tolerance with certainty. Based on our exercise times we can't talk of tolerance, because we didn't see a difference between initial testing and follow-up testing. Based on the blood pressure and heart rate changes there appears to be some tolerance.
Both during the initial testing and 5 months later, patients on nitrates were able to exercise for a longer time before they developed angina and ST-segment depression.

DISTANTE:

Would you please comment on possible mechanisms to explain the difference between partial tolerance, haemodynamic tolerance and antianginal effect?

DANAHY:

I believe that using our protocol, the blood pressure and heart rate changes are probably a more sensitive measure of the nitrate effect, than the antianginal effect. Personally, I assume that there is some tolerance to the antianginal effect as well but we were not able to demonstrate this with our protocol.
We could, however, demonstrate some tolerance to the heart rate and blood pressure changes.

DEMARIA:

Were heart rate and blood pressure measured at rest, and not during exercise? Under which condition did the blunting of heart rate and blood pressure response occur?

DANAHY:

On nitrates the end-exercise heart rate was higher but the end-exercise systolic pressure was generally the same, while the double product was larger at the end of exercise after medication, as compared to control values.
We didn't find any blunting of the blood pressure response at maximal exercise, only at rest.

FRANCIOSA:

It is obvious that defining tolerance depends on the parameters measured. Blood pressure is regulated by many mechanisms. I am not sure that blood pressure changes may be indicative of true tolerance. When blood pressure drops, many mechanisms come into play to restore it. Have you seen any changes in weight over several months in your patients? The initial hypotension may have caused fluid retention, and this cannot be regarded as true tolerance either.

DANAHY:

We did not measure weight at initial and follow-up testing. There was one patient who developed mild congestive heart failure during the course of the study, but he was the only patient in whom there was a detectable change. He was digitalized at that point.

Tolerance in Patients with Coronary Heart Disease Under Chronic Treatment with Isosorbide Dinitrate?

H.-J. Becker, R. Meudt, S. Kretschmer, H. D. Hüwer

The phenomenon of tolerance was described for the first time by Stewart in 1888 (32, 33). He wrote about a patient, in whom it took 20 grains of nitroglycerin to produce the same hypotensive effect as was initially achieved with 1/100 grain. Subsequently, a number of reports were published concerning the diminishing effects of nitrates during chronic treatment in respect to heart rate, blood pressure, and headache (5, 11, 12, 30, 35). On the other hand, withdrawal symptoms after chronic use of nitrates were seen (15, 27). The experiences with workers in dynamite factories are well known (9, 17, 20, 34). Definitions of tolerance, tachyphylaxis, and so on are given in Table 1. The main problem in chronic treatment with nitrates is whether tolerance occurs or not. We have carried out three studies and started a fourth with a view to providing an answer to this question.

The first study was undertaken in 1976 (4). Ten patients with coronary heart disease, angina, and reproducible ischemic ST-segment depression under exercise were treated over a period of 9 weeks with 30–100 mg isosorbide dinitrate (ISDN) daily. During that time repeated exercise tests were done before and after 10 mg or 30 mg ISDN or placebo. The investigation was done in double-blind manner. The different dosages of ISDN and placebo were randomized. The time between the last usual dosage and the tests was 6 h. The second exercise test after application of placebo or ISDN was performed 45 min after application. The patients data and results are shown in Tables 2–3 and Fig. 1.

Under these conditions we could see no signs of tolerance with respect to the parameter of ischemic ST-segment depression under exercise.

In a second study, 21 patients with coronary heart disease and reproducible ST-segment depression under exercise, who had been treated with ISDN in a dosage of 60–160 mg daily for 1½–9 years, were investigated. We performed exercise tests before and after

Table 1. Definitions of terms

Tachyphylaxis	Attenuation of the effect of a drug within minutes
Tolerance	Attenuation of antianginal effect or heart rate changes within weeks or months of chronic treatment; need to increase dosage to achieve the same effect during treatment or after the acute application of the drug
Partial tolerance	Absence of heart rate or blood pressure changes under chronic treatment, while antianginal effect remains present
Cross-tolerance	Decrease in antianginal effect of nitroglycerin during treatment with isosorbide dinitrate
Pseudotolerance	Counterregulation
Withdrawal phenomenon	Angina, myocardial infarction, or sudden death after abrupt discontinuatin of nitrate therapy
Dependence	Headache, angina or myocardial infarction during drug-free interval

Table 2. Patients of the first study

Patient	Sex	Age (years)	Workload		Duration (minutes)	Diagnosis			Angiographic pattern number of vessels with obstruction more than 50%
			mkp/s/ 1.73 sm	watts		angina pectoris	myocardial inferior	infarction apex	
1	Male	74	4	50	6	Yex	+	−	−
2	Male	50	4	50	3	Yes	−	−	3
3	Male	53	10	140	6	Yes	+ non transmural		3
4	Male	51	7	100	6	Yes	+		3
5	Male	54	7	125	5	Yes	−	−	2
6	Male	63	5	85	3	Yes	−	−	3
7	Female	63	4	40	5	Yes	+	−	3
8	Male	53	8	130	5	Yes	−	−	3
9	Male	54	8	120	3	Yes	−	−	3
10	Male	59	6	70	4	Yes	+ (and posterior)		−

Table 3. Sum of ST-segment depression (mm) under exercise in ten patients during st and 3rd (I), 3rd and 6th (II) and 6th and 9th (III) week of therapy with isosorbide dinitrate (ISDN)

Patient No.	Control			Placebo			10 mg ISDN			30 mg ISDN		
	I	II	III	I	II	III	I	II	III	I	II	III
1	14.9	15	11.2	14.9	6.5	16.8	10.8	2.5	6.5	3.1	2.7	3.1
2	5.9	14.2	3	5.7	7.1	1.6	5.5	5.4	1.1	4.8	5.6	0.7
3	8.8	16.5	9.3	7.3	7	9	9.4	9.3	6.1	9.8	3.6	3.4
4	2.4	5.2	2.5	3	2.9	2.5	1.9	2.5	3.1	1.4	1.6	0.7
5	11.2	7.7	14.1	10.1	7.3	6.9	1.4	2.2	3.8	1.3	6.3	1.9
6	7.2	12.5	5.5	9.4	2.9	6.3	6.3	3	1.1	1.8	1.8	0.8
7	4.7	6.9	4.9	2.9	6.3	2.1	3.1	2.6	2.7	1.1	3.8	1.2
8	4.6	8.6	4.5	5.2	3.5	5.9	4.6	2.8	5.2	4.8	2.3	2
9	7.5	14.2	9.4	5.2	11.1	7.4	4.2	4	6.7	1.1	2.6	3.1
10	5.8	2.5	3.7	3	2.1	3.5	3.1	0.9	2	0.8	0.9	1.5
$\bar{x}$	8.3	6.6	6.4	6.5	5.7	6.2	5	3.5	3.8	3	3.1	1.9
SE	1.5	1.1	1.2	1.2	0.9	1.4	1	0.7	0.7	0.9	0.5	0.3

Fig. 1. Nine weeks therapy with isosorbide dinitrate (ISDN) did not lead to tolerance. 10 and 30 mg ISDN given six hours after the usual dose achieved the same improvement during the first weeks of treatment (columns left) as after 9 weeks treatment (columns right)

Fig. 2. Patients, who were under chronic treatment with isosorbide dinitrate over a period of one and a half up to nine years did not show any signs of tolerance to a single dose of ISDN, concerning the interval of 24 hours between the last usual dose and the drug test.

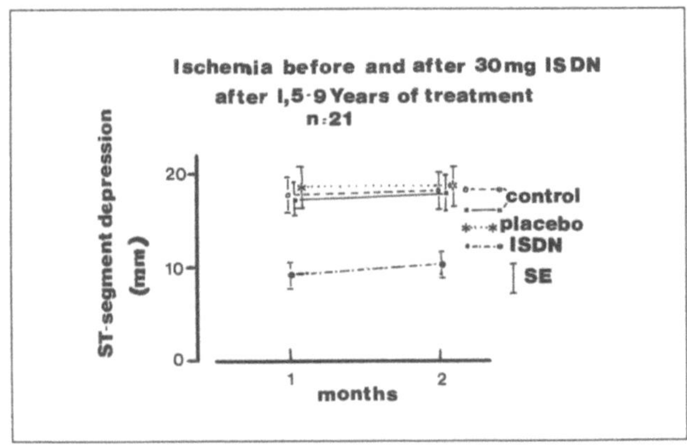

Fig. 3. Repeated exercise tests before and after 30 mg isosorbide dinitrate or placebo in patients, who are under chronic treatment with ISDN, revealed within six months no signs of tolerance.

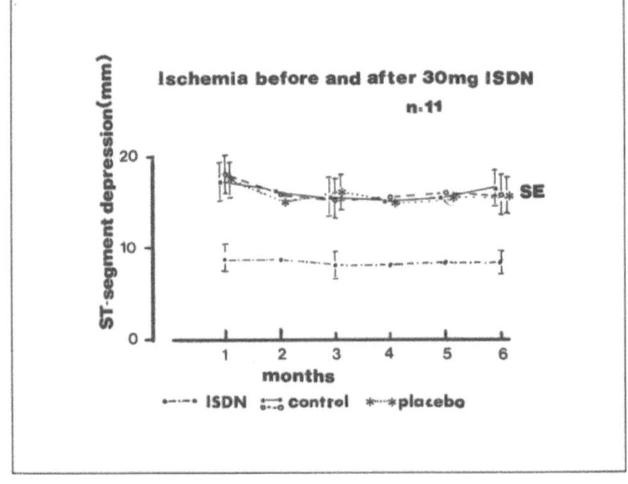

120

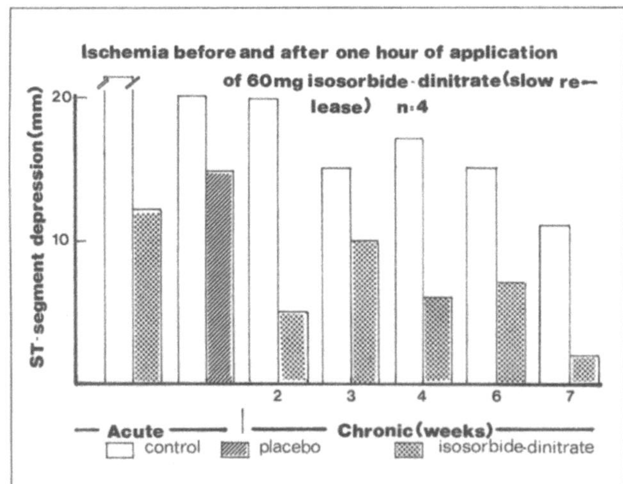

Fig. 4. Preliminary results of patients, who received 180–240 mg isosorbide dinitrate (slow released) showed no signs of tolerance within seven weeks of treatment. The response of ischemic ST-segment depression to ISDN (slow released) during exercise remained. The exercise tests were done before and one hour after the usual morning dose of slow released ISDN.

30 mg ISDN or placebo, which was given in a double-blind manner. The time between the last usual dosage and the tests was 24 h. The second exercise test was done 30 min after application of either 30 mg ISDN or placebo. The tests were repeated 2 months later. The patients data and results are shown in Tables 4–6 and Fig. 2. Some of the patients had taken slow-release or normal ISDN for a period of some years. None of the patients showed signs of tolerance in respect to ischemic ST-segment depression under exercise.

In a third investigation 11 patients with coronary heart disease and reproducible ST-segment depression under exercise, who were taking 60–160 mg ISDN daily, were observed over a period of 6 months. During that time, every month exercise tests were performed before and 30 min after 30 mg ISDN or placebo in a double-blind fashion. The exercise tests were performed after a 24-h interruption of the usual medication. Each patient underwent four exercise tests per month and 24 exercise tests over a period of 6 months. The patients data and results are shown in Table 7–8 and Fig. 3. We could see no signs of tolerance with respect either to ischemic ST-segment depression under exercise or to heart rate.

In a fourth study, which is running now, patients under 180–240 mg slow-release ISDN are being investigated. The patients have an exercise test before their usual morning dose and 1 and 3 h after they have taken 60 mg slow-release ISDN or placebo. The last usual dose is taken 8–12 h before, so the normal rhythm of application of the tablets is not interrupted. We have repeated the investigations every week for a period of 8 weeks. The results are shown in Fig. 4. These are preliminary data of four patients. Although the variance from the control tests is considerable, there is no sign of tolerance.

Tolerance has been discussed for more than 90 years. Arguments for tolerance were diminishing headaches and less acute heart rate changes under chronic treatment with nitrates even after a few days (5, 11, 12, 22, 30, 31). Many authors argued that in spite of partial tolerance the response of angina to nitrates would not be attenuated (3, 10, 12, 13, 14, 16, 18, 24). But some patients did report a decreased effect after longterm treatment. We saw in some cases a progression of coronary sclerosis as a cause for a diminished effect of nitrates. Our study of 1976 (4) showed no signs of tolerance.

Table 4. Patients of the second study

Patient	Sex	Age (years)	Workload		Duration (minutes)	Diagnosis			Angiographic pattern (number of vessels involved with obstruction more than 50%)
			mkp/s/ 1.73 sm	watts		Angina pectoris	old inferior	infarction apex	
1	Male	53	8	122	6	Yes	+	−	2
2	Male	52	8	108	4	Yes	−	−	2
3	Male	47	8	112	5	Yes	−	−	2
4	Male	44	12	198	5	Yes	−	+	2
5	Male	63	6	100	4	Yes	+	−	3
6	Male	47	6	80	3	Yes	+	−	3
7	Male	59	8	100	6	Yes	+	−	3
8	Female	54	6	70	5	Yes	−	+	3
9	Male	49	8	120	6	Yes	−	−	2
10	Male	54	6	85	3	Yes	−	−	3
11	Male	62	6	90	5	Yes	+	−	3
12	Male	61	6	90	5	Yes	−	−	3
13	Male	62	6	82	3	Yes	+	−	3
14	Male	53	8	122	3	Yes	+	−	3
15	Male	57	8	112	5	Yes	−	−	3
16	Male	36	10	148	6	Yes	−	−	3
17	Male	53	10	161	6	Yes	+	−	2
18	Male	60	8	113	5	Yes	−	−	3
19	Male	54	8	113	6	Yes	−	−	2
20	Male	67	8	112	6	Yes	−	+	2
21	Male	43	8	120	6	Yes	−	−	1

Table 5. Duration of therapy with isosorbide dinitrate (ISDN)

Patient no.	Preparation	Dose (mg/day)	Duration of ISDN therapy (years)
1	Isoket retard	120	$2^{1}/_{2}$
2	Isoket	60	2
3	Isoket	60	2
4	Maycor	80	3
5	Isoket retard	120	9
6	Isoket retard	80	8
7	Isomack retard forte	160	2
8	Isoket	160	7
9	Isoket	60	6
10	Isoket retard	120	5
11	Isoket retard	160	3
12	Isoket retard	80	7
13	Isoket retard	120	2
14	Isoket retard	160	2
15	Maycor	60	$3^{1}/_{2}$
16	Isoket	80	$1^{3}/_{4}$
17	Isoket	60	2
18	Isoket retard	120	2
19	Isoket retard	120	$1^{3}/_{4}$
20	Isomack retard	80	9
21	Isoket	80	$1^{1}/_{2}$
$\bar{x}$		102	3,9

Nowadays tolerance is again being discussed in Germany after the investigations of Blasini (6, 7). It has to be stated that second and third studies were made after a 24-h interval in the usual treatment with nitrates. When we planned the study we thought that tolerance might be caused by enzyme induction in the liver, which was discussed by Needleman and co-workers (28). This is not reversible in 24 h, but Blasini et al. (6, 7) reported that tolerance disappears after a 24-h interval without medication.

The reason for tolerance may be biochemical. It is possible that nitrate reacts with a reduced sulfhydryl group to form a disulfide linkage in the vascular receptor, the chemically altered receptor then being no longer responsive to nitrates (29). This might explain the attenuation of headaches after some days of treatment with nitrates. Whether this is due to a counterregulation is not yet known. Withdrawal symptoms have been reported by dynamite workers and patients (17, 19, 23, 25, 26, 34). We have seen a few patients who developed angina after abrupt cessation of nitrates; in one case sudden death occurred after a 24-h medication-free interval. In the literature there are many reports in which tolerance under chronic treatment with nitrates did not occur (1–4, 14, 16, 21, 36). There was no cross-tolerance between chronic oral application of ISDN and sublingually administered nitroglycerin either (12, 21, 22, 35). Some authors reported an attenuation of changes in blood pressure and heart rate under chronic treatment with nitrates, but it must be borne in mind, that these changes of heart rate, for example, are slight (less than 10%), and so insufficient to prove the phenomenon of tolerance.

Probably selection of patients plays a major role in this controversial area of investigation. Only patients with reproducible ST-segment depression during exercise were includ-

Table 6. ST-segment depression (mm) before and 30 minutes after 30 mg isosorbide dinitrate after 1.5–9 years of treatment in the 1st month (I) and 1 month later (II)

Patient No.	Control		Placebo		30 mg ISDN	
	I	II	I	II	I	II
1	12.5	14	14.5	14.5	8	7.5
2	15.5	16.5	15	16.5	7	11
3	12.5	11.5	12.5	9.5	6	5.5
4	9	11.5	9	9.5	4	3.5
5	44.5	47.5	50	51.5	27.5	28.5
6	27	28	29	31	17	16
7	11	10.5	12.5	12	7.5	6
8	28	31	32	30	18	16
9	12	14.5	13.5	19	7.5	11
10	23.5	26	26.5	29	12.5	21
11	15.5	12	14	9.5	5	5.5
12	13.5	14	14.5	13	4	6
13	21	20.5	20.5	21	15	15.5
14	26	24	30	26.5	14.5	16.5
15	13	10.5	12	11.5	4	4.5
16	13.5	14	14.5	13	4	6
17	14	15	12	16	8	11
18	15	16.5	14	18	4.5	12
19	24	25	23	22	14	12
20	13	14.5	10	14	4	4.5
21	10.5	9	14	9	3.5	2.5
$\bar{x}$	17.8	18.4	18.7	18.9	9.3	10.6
SE	1.9	2.0	2.2	2.2	1.4	1.4

ed in our studies but not in those of Rudolph (6, 7). It is well known that some patients with angina have a great variation in working capacity. These patients are not suitable candidates for drug studies because spontaneous variations can not be distinguished from the effects of the drug.

We prefer patients with safe reproducible ischemic reaction under exercise. No other medication is allowed during the drug tests.

Drug tests are of use if the following considerations apply:

1. Coronary sclerosis has been demonstrated.
2. Typical angina has been diagnosed.
3. Reproducible ST-segment depression occurs under exercise with same workload and duration.
4. Symptom-limited exercise tests are not carried out. (We prefer repeated exercise tests with the same workload and duration, leading to an ischemic pattern in the control test.)
5. No other medication is given. We discontinue digoxin 2 weeks and beta-blockers or calcium antagonists 48 h before the tests.
6. Placebo tests and controls after interruption of treatment are carried out.
7. ST-segment depression is measured during exercise and during a 3- or 5-min recovery period.

124

Table 7. Patients of the third study

Patient	Sex	Age (years)	Workload		Duration (minutes)	Diagnosis			Angiographic pattern (number of vessels involved with obstruction more than 50%)
			mkp/s/ 1.73 sm	watts		Angina pectoris	old inferior	infarction apex	
1	Male	60	8	116	5	Yes	–	–	3
2	Male	53	8	125	3	Yes	–	–	3
3	Male	54	8	120	6	Yes	+	–	2
4	Male	42	8	120	6	Yes	–	–	1
5	Male	62	6	88	3	Yes	+	–	3
6	Male	53	10	160	6	Yes	+	–	2
7	Male	62	6	97	5	Yes	+	–	3
8	Male	57	8	116	5	Yes	–	–	3
9	Male	61	6	78	5	Yes	–	–	3
10	Male	35	10	150	6	Yes	–	–	3
11	Male	47	8	116	5	Yes	+	–	2

Table 8. ST-segment depression (mm) over six months (n = 11)

Month of treat-ment	Control I		Control II		Placebo		Isosorbide-dinitrate (ISDN)		ISDN/ Placebo
	$\bar{x}$	SE	$\bar{x}$	SE	$\bar{x}$	SE	$\bar{x}$	SE	p-values
1	18.1	2.1	17.2	2.2	17.4	1.9	8.8	1.6	0.003
2	16	2.4	16.1	2	15.1	1.9	8.6	1.6	0.003
3	15.4	2.3	15.6	2.2	16	2.1	8.1	1.6	0.003
4	15.6	2.2	15.1	2.2	15.1	2.1	7.9	1.5	0.003
5	16.1	2.4	15.6	2.1	15.9	2	8.5	1.6	0.003
6	15.9	2.3	16.6	2.1	15.8	2.2	8.5	1.4	0.003

It is true, that this selection cannot be representative for all patients with coronary heart disease, but the effectiveness of antianginal drugs can only be studied under clearly defined conditions because these patients often show great variability of symptoms.

References

1. Abrams J: Nitrate tolerance and dependence. Amer Heart J Vol 99, 1 S. 113–122 (1980).
2. Abrams J: Nitrate tolerance and dependence. La Nouvelle Presse Medicale 9, No. 34 S. 2499–2504 (1980).
3. Aronow WS, Chesluk HM: Evaluation of nitroglycerin in angina in patients on isosorbide dinitrate. Circulation 42: 61–63 (1970).
4. Becker HJ, Walden G, Kaltenbach M: Gibt es eine „Tachyphylaxie" bzw. Gewöhnung bei der Behandlung der Angina pectoris mit Nitrokörpern? Verh Dtsch Ges Inn Med 82. Bd. 1208–1210, J. F. Bergmann München 1976.
5. Bernstein LM, Ivy AC: Inositol and mannitol hexanitrates in hypertensive management. Circulation 12: 353 (1955).
6. Blasini R, Brügmann U, Mannes A, Froer KL, Hall D, Rudolph W: Wirksamkeit von ISDN in retardierter Form bei Langzeitbehandlung. Herz 5: 298–305 (1980).
7. Blasini R, Brügmann U, Froer KL, Fleck E, Rudoph W: Gibt es eine Toleranzentwicklung bei oraler Langzeitbehandlung mit Nitraten? Verh Dtsch Ges Inn Med Bd. 88, J. F. Bergmann München 1982, im Druck.
8. Brunner D, Weisbord J, Meshulam N, Margulis S: Langzeitwirkung und Dauertherapie mit kutan appliziertem ISDN bei Patienten mit koronarer Herzkrankheit. Münch Med Wschr 122: 21, 801–806 (1980).
9. Carmichel P, Lieben J: Sudden death in explosives workers. Arch Environ Health 7: 50–54 (1963).
10. Chandraratna PAN, Langevin E, O'Dell R, Rubinstein C, San Pedro S: Use of nitroglycerin ointment in congestive heart failure. Cardiology 63: 337–339 (1978).
11. Crandall LA, Leake CD, Loevenheart AS, Mühlberger CW: Acquired tolerance to and cross tolerance between the nitrous and nitric acid esters and sodium nitrite in man. 3. Pharmacol Exp Ther 41: 103–120 (1931).
12. Danahy DT, Aronow WS: Hemodynamics and antianginal effects of high dose oral ISDN after chronic use. Circulation 56: 205–212 (1977).
13. Franciosa JA, Miculic E, Cohn JN, Jose E, Fabie A: Hemodynamic effects of orally administered ISDN in patients with congestive heart failure. Circulation 50: 1020–1024 (1974).
14. Franciosa JA, Cohn JN: Sustained hemodynamic effects of nitrates without tolerance in heart failure. Circulation 57/58: S. 11–28 (1978).
15. Franciosa JA, Nordstrom LA, Cohn JN: Nitrate therapy for congestive heart failure. D Amer Med Ass 240: 443 (1978).

16. Goldstein RE, Rosing DR, Redwood DR, Beiser GD, Epstein SE: Clinical and circulatory effects of isosorbide dinitrate. Comparison with nitroglycerin. Circulation 43: 629–640 (1971).
17. Klock JC: Nonocclusive coronary disease after chronic exposure to nitrates: evidence for physiologic nitrate dependence. Amer Heart J 89: 510 (1975).
18. Kovick RB, Tillisch JH, Berens SC, Bramowitz AD, Shine KI: Vasodilator therapy of chronic left ventricular failure. Circulation 53: 322 (1976).
19. Lange RL, Reid MS, Tresch DD, Keelan MH, Bernhard VM, Collidge G: Non-atheromatous ischemic heart disease following withdrawal from chronic industrial nitroglycerin exposure. Circulation 46: 666 (1972).
20. Laws GC: The effects of nitroglycerin upon those who manufacture it. Am Med Ass 21: 793 (1898).
21. Lee G, Mason DT, DeMaria AN: Effects of long-term oral administration of isosorbide dinitrate on the antianginal response to nitroglycerin. Amer J Cardiol 41: 82–87 (1978).
22. Lichtlen PR: Langzeitnitrate bei Angina pectoris. Münch Med Wschr 122: 49, 1753–1754 (1980).
23. Lund RP, Haggendahl J, Johnsson G: Withdrawal symptoms in workers exposed to nitroglycerine. Br J Inn Med 25: 136 (1968).
24. Massie B, Chatterjee K, Werner J, Greenberg B, Hart R, Parmley WW: Hemodynamic advantage of combined administration of hydralazine orally and nitrates nonparenterally in the vasodilator therapy of chronic heart failure. Amer J Cardiol 40: 794–801 (1977).
25. Morikawa Y, Muraki K, Ikoma Y, Honda T, Takamatsu H: Organic nitrate poisoning at an explosives factory. Arch Environ Health 7: 50 (1963).
26. Morton WE: Occupational habituation to aliphatic nitrates and the withdrawal hazards of coronary disease and hypertension. J Occup Med 19: 197 (1977).
27. Muller J, Gunther SJ: Nifedipine therapy for Prinzmetal's angina. Circulation 57: 737 (1978).
28. Needleman P, Hunter FE: The transformation of glyceryl trinitrate and other nitrates by glutathione organic nitrate reductase. Molec Pharmacol 1: 77–86 (1965).
29. Needleman P, Johnson EM: Mechanism of tolerance development organic nitrates. J Pharm Exp Ther 184: 709–715 (1973).
30. Schelling JL, Lasagna L: A study of cross tolerance to circulatory effects of organic nitrates. Clin pharm Ther 8: 256–260 (1967).
31. Shane SJ, Iazetta JJ, Chisholm AW, Berka JF, Leung D: Plasma concentrations of isosorbide dinitrate and its metabolites after chronic oral dosage in man. Brit J clin pharmacol 6: 37–41 (1978).
32. Stewart DD: Remarkable tolerance to nitroglycerine. Philadelphia Polyclinic, 1888, 172.
33. Stewart DD: Tolerance to nitroglycerine. J amer med ass 44: 1678–1679 (1905).
34. Symanski H: Schwere Gesundheitsschädigungen durch berufliche Nitroglykoleinwirkung. Arch Hyg Bakt 136: 139 (1952).
35. Thadani V, Manyari D, Parker JD, Fung H: Tolerance to the circulatory effects of oral isosorbide dinitrate. Rate of development and cross tolerance to glyceryl trinitrate. Circulation 61: 526–535 (1980).
36. Winsor W, Berger HJ: Oral nitroglycerin as a prophylactic antianginal drug: Clinical, physiologic and statistical evidence of efficacy based on a threephase experimental design. Amer Heart J 90: 611–626 (1975).
37. Zelis R, Mason DT: ISDN, effect on the vasodilator response to nitroglycerin. JAMA, 234: 166–170 (1975).

Author adress:
Prof. Dr. H.-J. Becker
Medizinische Klinik I
Stadtkrankenhaus
Leimenstraße 20
D-6450 Hanau 1

Discussion

KALTENBACH:

Except for your very last study, your results refer to situations in which, apparently, the effect of the chronic ISDN administration had subsided at the time you started your investigations. One could possibly argue that these results are those of an intermittent ISDN therapy.

BECKER:

I agree in principle, but if you look at the first study we did in 1976, there was an interval of 6 hours only between the end of the long term therapy and the start of the investigation. This is the usual dose interval patients keep anyway. I therefore believe we thus imitated the normal dose regimen with a six hours' interval. Your criticism is correct for the second and third study where we interrupted the treatment over a period of 24 hours. When we started these studies we thought that tolerance could be abolished within 24 hours, but rather a longer interruption of treatment. We now started again with the sustained-release formulation of ISDN to imitate the normal treatment: The patients received normal ISDN tablets until 9 p.m., and on the next morning we started the first test before they took their usual dose. We then repeated the testing one and 3 hours later respectively.

KALTENBACH:

I agree with you that your first study design corresponded to the normal nitrate regimen. On the other hand, exercise testing with placebo during the long term therapy yielded the same results as the first placebo test. Wouldn't that mean that chronic treatment, at the time of re-testing, was no longer effective, in other words, with your study design, the single dose was effective for less than six hours? At the end of that time interval you renewed the dose for another six hours, and so on....

BECKER:

That is possible, but I do not know the reason for possibly developing tolerance. I do not know whether it is due to receptor blockade. If this were so, the blockade should persist for more than 6 hours.

KENEDI:

We conducted a study with a design similar to that reported by Dr. Rudolph at the Monte Carlo Meeting. So far, we have preliminary results in 4 patients. In these 4 patients, we didn't find any significant enhancement of the ST-segment depression after 4 weeks' treatment.

BECKER:

My discussion with Dr. Rudolph in Venice in November 1981 about this problem has shown that one reason for his results was that he did not look for reproducible ST-segment depressions. If the reproducibility of the ST-segment depression during exercise in patients with coronary heart disease is not investigated, highly variable ST-segment depressions may be found. This variability depends on the climate and on other special problems. The other point is that some of the patients were treated for a long time with betablockers, and the interval between the last dose and exercise testing was 12 hours only, so that at that time (12 hours) an effect of the beta blockade should be expected to persist.

WOODCOCK:

I would like to make some remarks to Dr. Becker's definition of tolerance and also the interaction of nitrates with the sulfhydryl groups in the so-called receptors. This definition would correspond to a pharmacodynamic model, but tolerance might also be due to a change in pharmacokinetics.

BECKER:

In principle, I agree, but there are many studies published in the literature where the problem of kinetics has been investigated. We know that the absorption is very good and there are high levels of metabolites. The kinetic data don't show any changes of absorption or an increase of metabolism or excretion.

FOX:

I should tike to comment on the ST-segment depression. This parameter shows how many millimeters of ST-segment depression there are before and after an intervention. But there is not a single shred of evidence that the ST-segment depression in one or many leads or the amount of ST-segment depression reflects the severity or extent of myocardial ischemia. If they are related, are they related directly or exponentially?

FRANCIOSA:

I would like to underline that ST-segments are not affected by nitrates only, but by many other factors. Thus, severe nitrate-induced tachycardia could worsen ST-segment depression, and this might be called tolerance, but it would actually be a very potent effect of the drug.

BECKER:

The behaviour of the ST-segment during exercise seems to be a better parameter than the amount of nitroglycerin consumption or subjective information, such as number and severity of anginal attacks.

DEMARIA:

Even though ST-segements changes may not be quantitatively related to ischaemia, I think everyone would agree that it is better to have less of ST-segment depression rather than more.

KOBER:

We have studied the correlation between ST-segment depression and the degree of coronary stenoses. We found a rather good correlation between the amount and the severity of the stenosis and the extent of poststenotic ischaemia. This however, depends on the site of the stenosis. If the stenosis is located in proximal parts of a coronary vessel, a larger ST-segment depression will be found. There is a good correlation, too, between ST-segment depression and myocardial function. A short question to Dr. Becker's third study: Did you find differences between patients treated with sustained release ISDN and those on normal tablets?

BECKER:

It is correct that in our third study patients were treated both with slow release and with normal tablets, but there was no difference. So, I couldn't answer the question whether a sustained release formulation causes tolerance more readily than normal tablets.

Long-Term Effects of High-Dose ISDN Therapy in Patients with Coronary Heart Disease

W. Schneider, B. Stahl, W. D. Bussmann, and M. Kaltenbach

The present study was designed to determine whether a dose-response relationship exists in the treatment of angina pectoris with oral isosorbide dinitrate (ISDN) and to investigate the possible development of tolerance to the antianginal effects of ISDN during therapy with 480 mg per day (see Fig. 1–4).

The study population comprised 11 male patients. All had stable angina due to angiographically proved coronary heart disease. Their ages ranged from 47 to 60 years (average 53 years). The study was designed in a single-blind manner. ISDN was administered orally six times a day using single doses of 5 mg, 20 mg, 40 mg, and 80 mg, thus attaining daily doses of 30 mg, 120 mg, 240 mg, and 480 mg. The sequence of the doses was randomized. Each dose level was maintained for 7 days during the first part of the trial. During this time only sublingual Nitroglycerin was permitted if necessary. The number of anginal attacks during treatment was recorded by the patients. On the final day of each phase of treatment an exercise stress test using an arm-assisted step test with a individually defined submaximum workload was performed 1 h after administration of ISDN. Exercise was terminated at a maximum of 6 min. The workload was determined in a separate test without medication prior to the study. Workload and exercise duration were held constant for each patient during the entire trial. The sum of ST-segment depression during

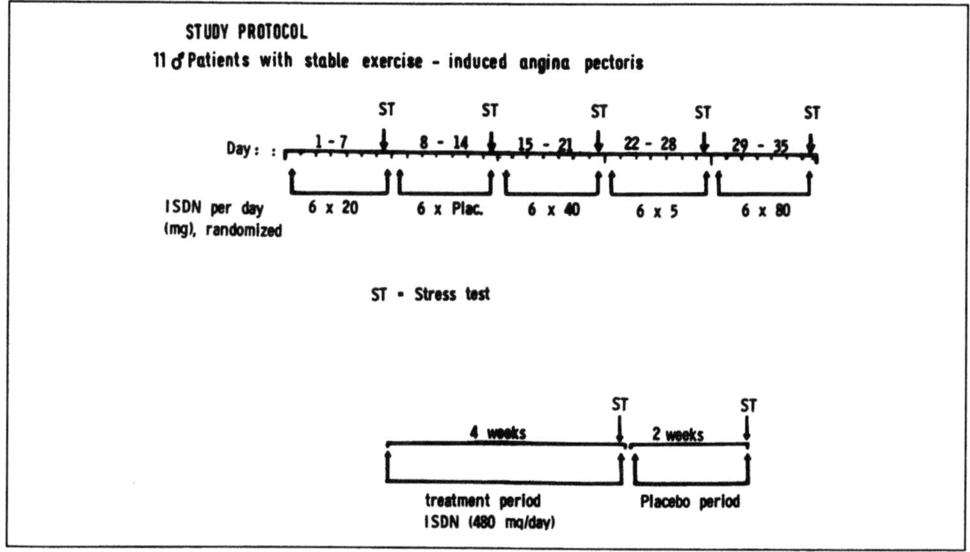

Fig. 1a,b. Study protocol: *ST,* stress test. a study population comprising 11 male patients (47–60) with stable exercise-induced angina, who were given varying doses of isosorbide dinitrate (*ISDN*) for 7 days each in a randomized sequence; b second trial: 480 mg ISDN per day for 4 weeks and second placebo period.

exercise and recovery was assessed. Blood pressure and heart rate were measured 1 h after the administration of ISDN. At the same time and 4 h after intake blood samples for the determination of ISDN and two metabolites were obtained.

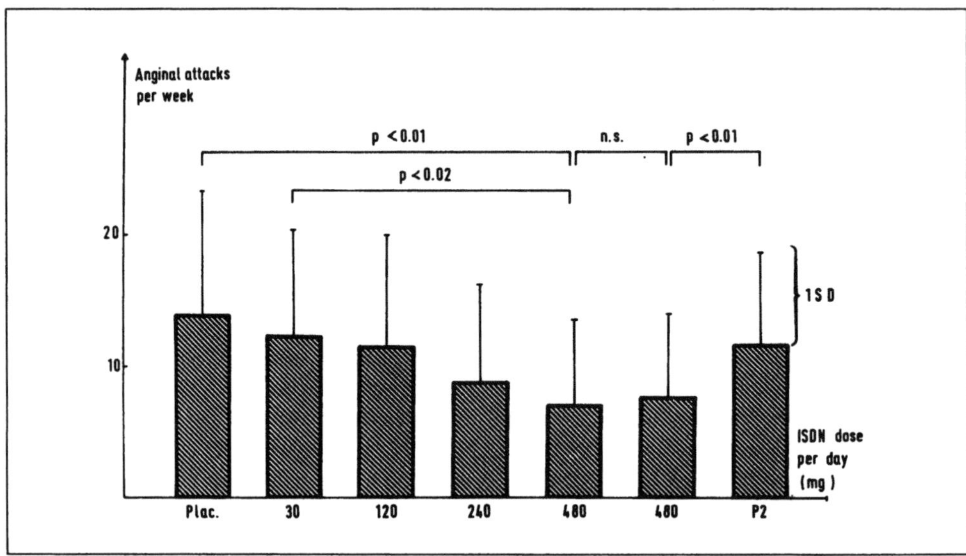

Fig. 2. Number of anginal attacks per week in patients with coronary heart disease after oral treatment with isosorbide dinitrate (*ISDN*) in varying dosages (mean ± SD). *P*, placebo.

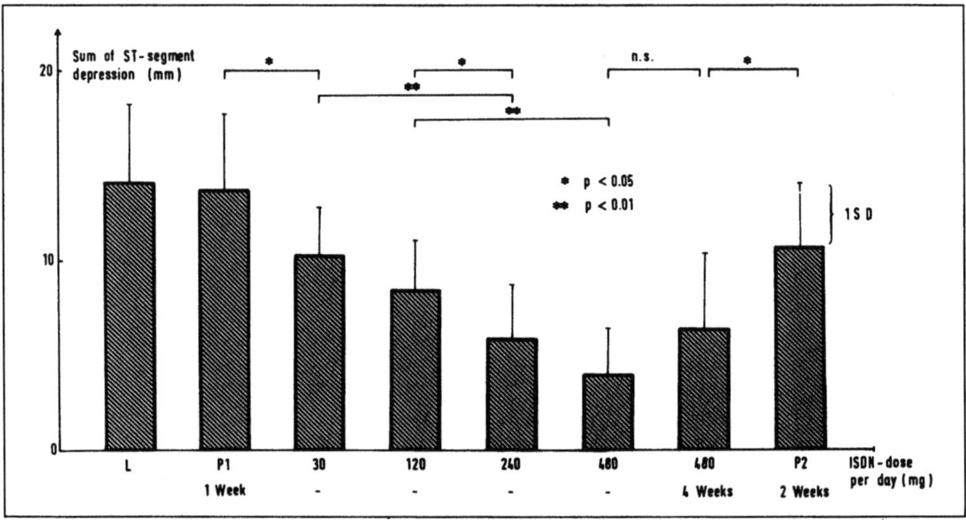

Fig. 3. Sum of ST-segment depression at the end of exercise stress testing in male patients with coronary heart disease after oral treatment with isosorbide dinitrate (*ISDN*) in varying dosages (mean ± SD). *P*, placebo; *$p < 0.05$; **$p < 0.02$; ***$p < 0.01$.

132

In a second trial, the patients continued therapy with 480 mg of ISDN per day for 4 weeks (Fig. 1b). After this time a stress test was performed in the same manner as described above. This was followed by a 2-week placebo period, at the end of which another stress test was performed. The results obtained are given in Fig. 2.

With increasing doses, a decline in the frequency of anginal attacks could be noted, being statistically significant between placebo and 480 mg and 30 mg and 480 mg ISDN. Thus the frequency of anginal attacks was reduced by 54% from 13.9 per week during the placebo period to 7.6 per week during the 1-week period with 480 mg. Continuation of the high-dose treatment did not lead to a significant loss of antianginal efficacy.

Figure 3 depicts the sum of ST-segment depression in the exercise tests. The mean sum of ST-segment depression decreased from 12.8 mm during the stress test without medication to 10.2 mm during the lowest ISDN phase (30 mg), and to 3.9 mm during the highest ISDN period (480 mg). During the following 4-week treatment period with 480 mg, the antianginal efficacy was slightly, but not statistically significant, attenuated (6.1 mm). A dose-related antianginal effect of oral ISDN is clearly shown. After 8 weeks of treatment, including a 5-week period with very high doses, no tolerance to the antianginal effects of the drug could be noted.

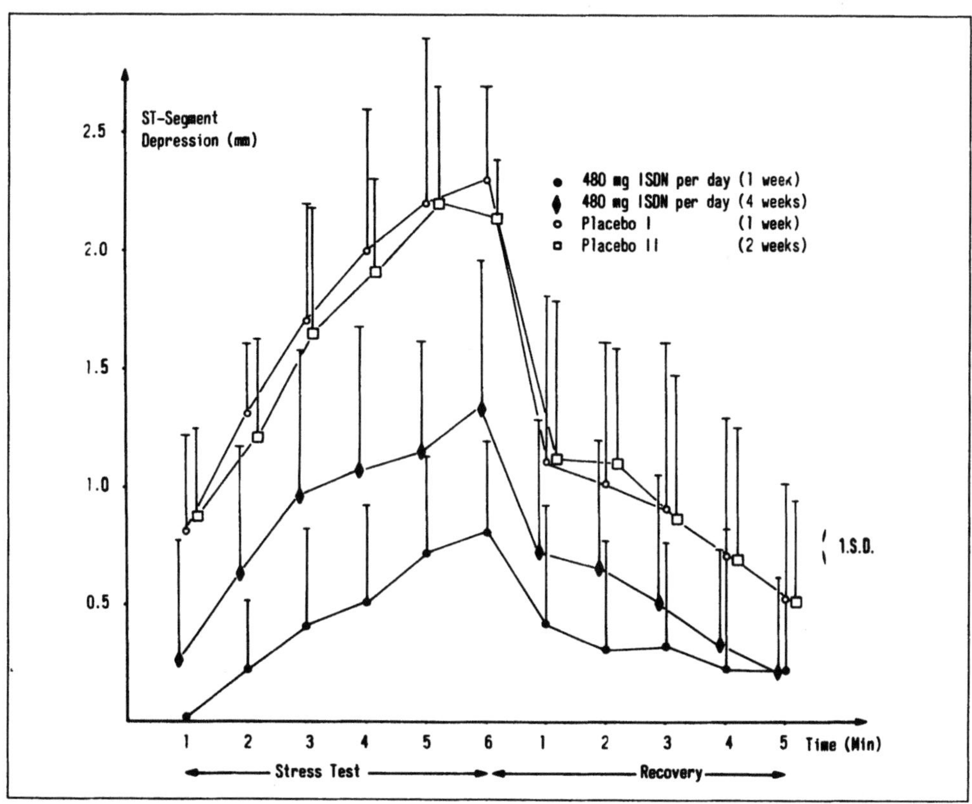

Fig. 4. ST-segment depression during exercise stress testing and recorvery (mean ± SD). *ISDN*, isosorbide dinitrate.

In Fig. 4 the data are illustrated in terms of ST-segment depression during each minute of stress testing and recovery. It can be seen that the results of the two placebo periods are nearly identical. The 4-week treatment period with 480 mg/day led to a moderate attenuation of the efficacy. The long-term efficacy of this dose corresponds to the potency of 120–240 mg after a 1-week period.

Figure 5 and table 1 show the plasma levels of ISDN and the mononitrates 1 and 4 h after administration of 5, 20, 40, and 80 mg of the drug. There is an almost linear increase in the plasma levels of ISDN and the mononitrates with increasing oral doses. The highest plasma levels were attained by isosorbide-5-mononitrate (837 ± 443 ng/ml). After a single oral dose of 40 or 80 mg of ISDN the parent compound itself exhibited considerable plasma levels (31 and 48 ng/ml·respectively). Four hours after ISDN application the plasma levels for the parent compound showed a greater decrease than those for the mononitrates according to the different plasma half-lives.

Figure 6 shows arterial blood pressure in the supine position directly before stress testing. With various doses of ISDN no significant change in blood pressure could be seen.

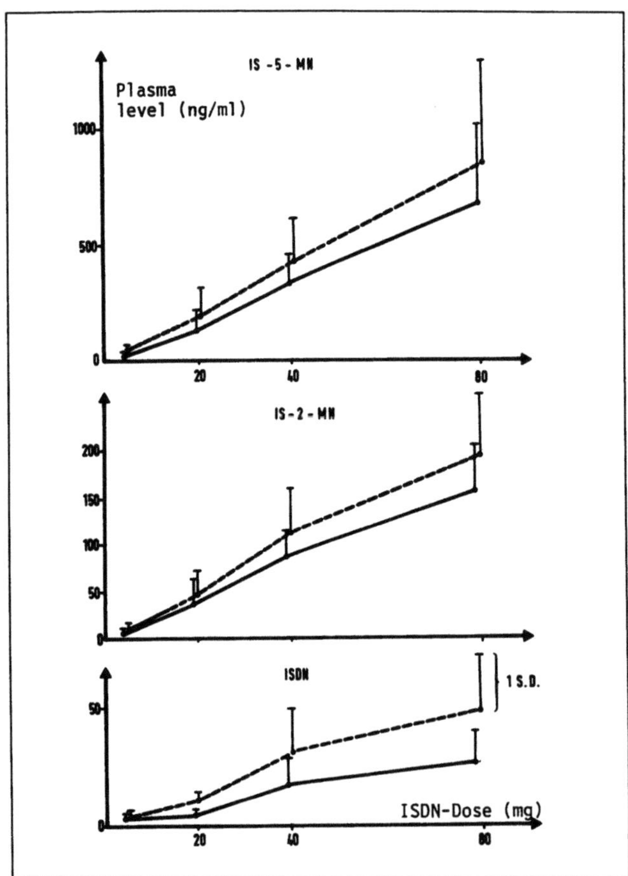

Fig. 5. Plasma levels of isosorbide dinitrate (*ISDN*), isosorbide-5-mononitrate (*IS-5-MN*), and isosorbide-2-mononitrate (*IS-2-MN*) in male patients with CHD (n = 11) one hour (O------O) and four hours (O————O) after oral intake of 5, 20, 40 and 80 mg ISDN.

Table 1.

Single dose	ISDN		IS-2-MN		IS-5-MN	
	1 h	4 h	1 h	4 h	1 h	4 h
5	3.2 ±1.9	1.3 ±0.7	10.8 ±4.3	4.9 ±2.9	47.2 ±20.1	25.2 ±15.5
20	9.8 ±5.5	4.5 ±3.5	48.3 ±26.8	38.7 ±29.3	191.6 ±124.2	131.5 ±91.1
40	31.7 ±18.8	17.4 ±11.5	113.3 ±48.1	88.1 ±30.3	424.8 ±193.3	332.8 ±129.7
80	48.3 ±24.0	26.6 ±13.68	194.7 ±66.5	156.8 ±50.3	837.7 ±443.2	670.4 ±346.1
	A	B	A	B	A	B

A: Determination one hour after administration
B: Determination four hours after administration

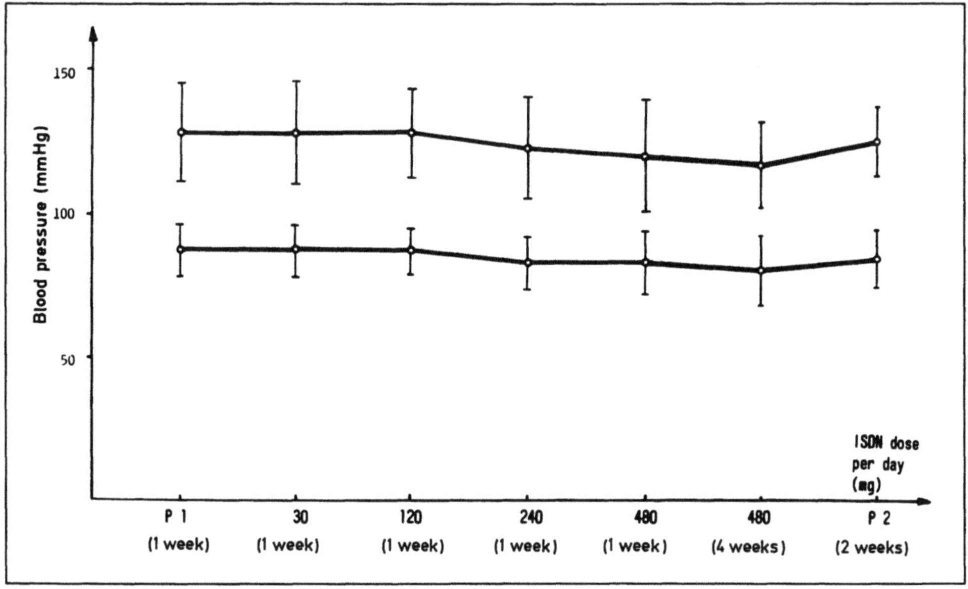

Fig. 6. Systolic and diastolic blood pressure in male patients with coronary heart disease after oral treatment with isosorbide dinitrate (*ISDN*) in varying dosages (mean ± SD). *P*, placebo.

Figure 7 shows heart rate at rest in the supine and in the standing position 1h after administration of the drug. This parameter showed a tendency to higher rates with increasing doses of ISDN, although these differences were not statistically significant. (The mean heart rate after a 1-week treatment period with 480 mg of ISDN in the standing position was 82 beats/min, and 86 beats/min and 77 beats/min following the 4-week treatment period with 480 mg/day and the 2-week placebo period respectively.)

Figure 8 shows heart rate during and after exercise-testing. Neither dosage nor time of treatment led to significant changes in heart rate during stress-testing. Mean maximum

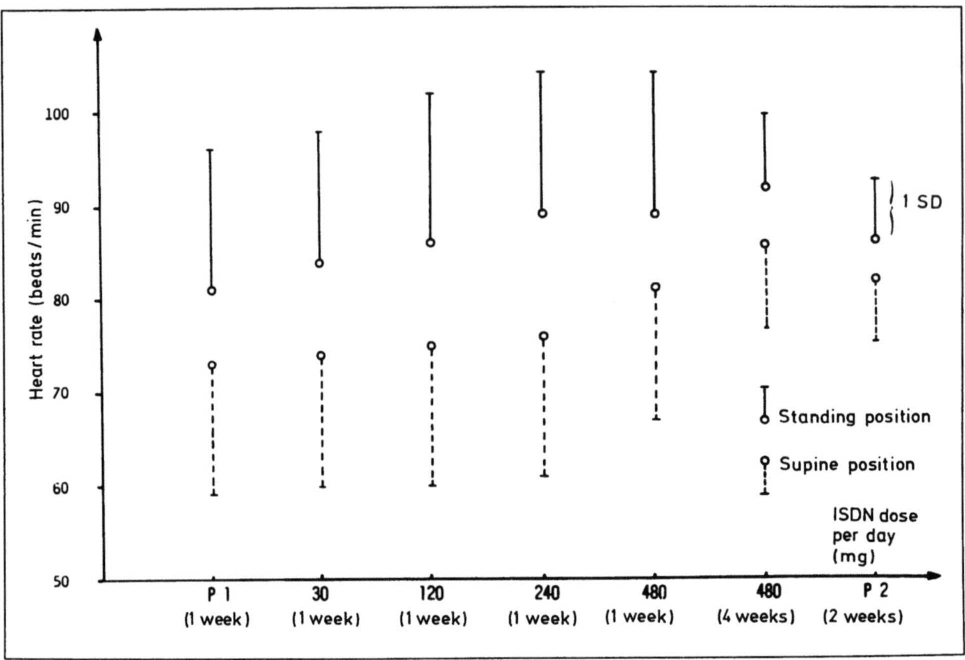

Fig. 7. Heart rate at rest in supine and standing position 1 h following drug administration in male patients with coronary heart disease after treatment with isosorbide dinitrate (*ISDN*) in varying dosages (mean ± SD). *P*, placebo.

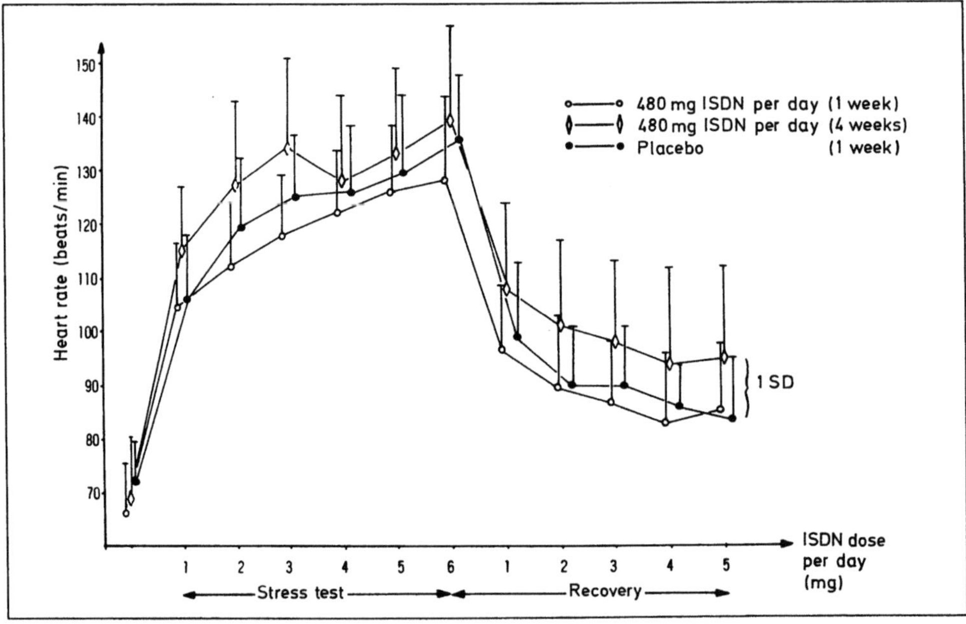

Fig. 8. Heart rate during and after exercise stress testing in male patients with coronary heart disease after high dosages of isosorbide dinitrate (*ISDN*) for varying periods.

136

heart rate after 1 week of treatment with 480 mg ISDN per day was 129/min compared to 139/min after 4 weeks of treatment and 137 beats/min after the placebo period.

The side-effects of the 8-week trial with various oral doses of ISDN (including a 5-week continuous treatment with 480 mg/day) were as follows:

1. Headache was present in five of eleven patients (54%) during 2–3 weeks of the initial treatment period of 5 weeks. Headache was initially more pronounced with higher dosages of ISDN.
   Headache was absent in all 11 patients undergoing additional treatment with 480 mg ISDN per day for 4 weeks.
2. Two of 11 patients reported signs of orthostatic dysregulation during the initial 5-week trial. These symptoms were absent during the 4-week high oral dosage treatment in all 11 patients.
3. One Patient complained of epigastric pain during the first treatment period.
4. Methemoglobin formation was below 1% during chronic high oral dosages of ISDN.

Summary:

1. The treatment of angina pectoris with oral ISDN resulted in a dose-dependent reduction of anginal attacks and a dose-related reduction of ischemic ST-segment depression.
2. Chronic oral treatment did not influence blood pressure at rest nor heart rate at rest and during exercise.
3. The plasma levels of ISDN and its metabolites exhibited a linear dose relationship with isosorbide-5-mononitrate showing the highest concentrations.
4. After 4 weeks of continuous treatment with 480 mg ISDN, a moderate attenuation but no significant reduction in antianginal efficacy could be observed.
   This result i.e. no reduction in antianginal activity after 4 week high dose ISDN treatment has been confirmed by a second study performed with a randomized, double blind protocol.

Authors' address:
Dr. W. Schneider
Zentrum der Inneren Medizin
Abteilung für Kardiologie
Klinikum der Universität
Theodor-Stern-Kai 7
6000 Frankfurt/Main 70

Discussion

FRANCIOSA:

Did you warn the patients prior to the start of medication that they might have headaches or did the patients spontaneously complain of headaches?

SCHNEIDER:

54% of the patients complained of headache during the first 2 to 3 days, but headache was not severe and there was no difficulty in continuing the treatment.
Most patients had already been on nitrates before and were familiar with nitrate headaches. Because of the nitrate-free interval (i.e. placebo period) it is understandable that some of the patients experienced headaches again when treatment was resumed.

DEMARIA:

We compared nitrates to placebo, and we instructed everyone that they might experience headaches, and the incidence of headaches in the placebo group was nearly as great as in the nitrate group.

SCHNEIDER:

We made similar observations. Some patients complained of headaches during the placebo period as well.

KALTENBACH:

I think there are quite a few double blind studies which clearly demonstrate that nitrates may, in a considerable number of patients, cause headaches. I would rather not question this. But I think that the disappearance of headaches during prolonged treatment is remarkable. This finding has been consistently reported in many studies. Apparently, partial tolerance does occur, but this does not necessarily mean tolerance to the antianginal effect.

DEMARIA:

I certainly agree that headaches occur from nitrates, but I just wonder about the frequency with which they are reported in various studies. Partially, that may be a negative placebo effect, depending on how the patient was advised prior to the medication.

FRANCIOSA:

We have done placebo-controlled studies with ISDN in heart failure, and the incidence of initial headaches was quite high in the nitrate group, but after 3 or 4 days, the incidence of headaches in the two groups was identical. In long-term therapy, there is no difference in the incidence of headaches.

KALTENBACH:

In view of the importance of investigation methods for tolerance problems I would like to take up again the matter of the ST-segment depression. This is a tool which may well be used. It is, however, important, in which way it is used. Under these particular circumstances, our design is different in two regards. The most important is probably that we do not use a symptom-limited type of exercise. If a symptom-limited type of exercise is used, variability is tied to the subjects' complaints, and ST-segment depression comes in second. All the variations derived from the subjectively experienced anginal pains are then interpreted in the light of the amount of ST-segment depression. If, on the other hand, one uses a type of exercise with exactly the same work-load and the same duration and if one looks at the ST-segment depression independently of subjective parameters, this is a far more useful tool. Doing it in this way, one can really show a dose-effect relationship.

FOX:

Of course I agree that ST-segment is an important tool for the assessment of antianginal efficacy in treatment, and I would agree that intuitively it is better to have less ST-segment depression than more and I would agree that there is a crude relationship between the arterial anatomy and the amount of ST-segment depression. Yet, improvement of ST-segment depression in the exercise ECG is not necessarily a measure of reduced ischaemia.

SCHNEIDER:

We indeed consider a standardized work-load with measurement of ST-segment depression to be the most objective parameter nowadays. In an experimental animal study ST-segments changes were compared to metabolic changes such as lactate accumulation and decrease in oxygen tension and good correlation was found between ST-segment and metabolic parameters.

DANAHY:

I think whether you demonstrate nitrate tolerance depends not only on how you look for it, but also when you look for it. Dr. Schneider compared the results obtained after one versus four weeks of therapy. Is it possible that already after one week some tolerance has developed? And therefore less tolerance could be found by comparing the end of the first week with the end of four weeks when comparing first-dose to 4 weeks findings?

BUSSMANN:

The first control was indeed, made after one week of treatment. Perhaps some tolerance had developed during this period. But the acute effect of 30 mg isosorbide dinitrate with a 50% reduction of ST-segment depression was about the same as after one week.

WOODCOCK:

I would like to ask for the meaning of the two curves in the lower figure of the ISDN serum levels.

SCHNEIDER:

The upper curve shows the plasma concentration 1 h after drug intake, and the lower curve represented by a dotted line, means the plasma level 4 hours after administration of ISDN.

Evaluation of Cross-Tolerance Between Long-Term Oral Isosorbide Dinitrate and Sublingual Nitroglycerin: Assessment by Exercise Testing

Anthony N. DeMaria; Garrett Lee, Reginald I. Low, Dean T. Mason,

Introduction

Recent studies have documented the ability of orally administered isosorbide dinitrate (ISDN), when administered in sufficiently large doses, to induce beneficial antianginal effects in patients with coronary artery disease (1–4). Accordingly, enhanced exercise tolerance, alleviation of symptoms, reduced electrocardiographic manifestations of myocardial ischemia, and favorable alterations in cardiocirculatory hemodynamics have all been demonstrated after the oral administration of ISDN (1–13). However, the question of whether or not chronic oral consumption of isosorbide induces tolerance to the nitrate effect remains unresolved. In particular, the ability of chronic oral isosorbide administration to abolish the acute response to sublingual nitroglycerin would have major implications regarding the application of this agent in patients with coronary disease. The issue of induction of tolerance to sublingually administered nitroglycerin by orally administered ISDN has assumed greater importance in view of the increased application of this agent in patients with ischemic heart disease in recent years. Therefere, we conducted a study to assess the effects of long-term oral administration of ISDN on the antianginal response to nitroglycerin by means of exercise stress testing.

Methods

Twenty-eight patients with the typical age and sex distribution of a coronary artery disease population were evaluated. All patients had stable angina pectoris, and coronary artery disease was confirmed in each patient who underwent arteriography. All cardiac medications were discontinued prior to study. Each of the patients had been documented to be a nitroglycerin responder in that they had previously manifested 1 mm or more ST-segment depression on electrocardiogram during treadmill exercise testing, and had subsequently responded to the sublingual administration of nitroglycerin with an increased duration of treadmill exertion.

Exercise stress testing was performed according to the protocol of Bruce et al. A motorized treadmill was utilized, electrocardiographic leads I, aVF, and V_5 were monitored continuously throughout the exercise test, and a full 12-lead electrocardiogram was performed prior to and at termination of exercise. Blood pressure was measured by cuff sphygmomanometer. Maximal exercise testing was performed to symptom-limited exertion. As previously stated, all patients had had prior exposure to this form of exercise testing to negate the effect of habituation on the reproducibility of exertional performance.

141

Fig. 1. Summary of the study protocol. *ET*, exercise test; *ISDN*, isosorbide dinitrate; dinitrate; *Max*, maximal symptom-limited exertion; *NTG*, nitroglycerin; *PO*, orally; *TID*, three times daily.

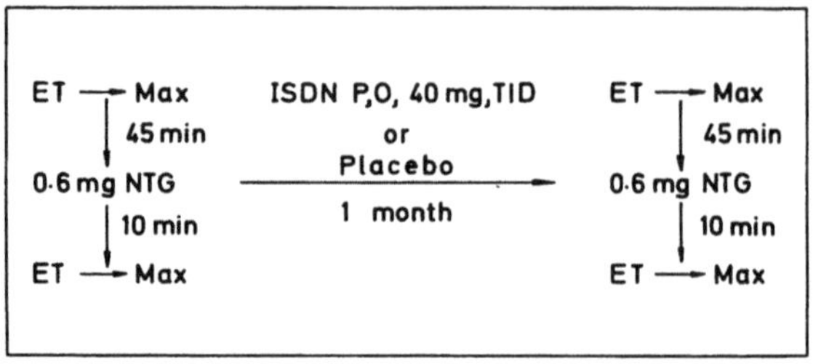

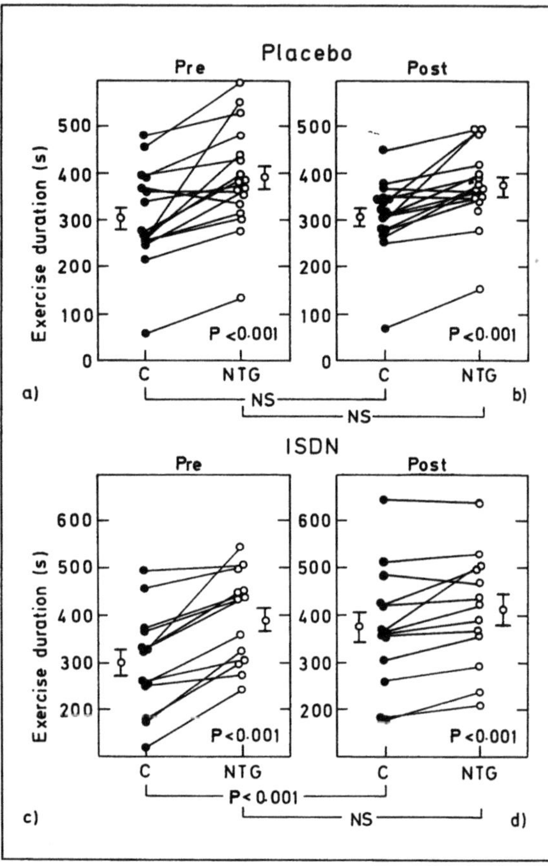

Fig. 2a–d. Individual, group mean, and SEM data for exercise duration before (*Pre*) and after (*Post*) 1 month of treatment with placebo or isosorbide dinitrate (*ISDN*) capsules. Prenitroglycerin control (*C*) and postnitroglycerin (*NTG*) exercise tests were performed at each period.

The protocol followed in this study is summarized in Fig. 1. At the initiation of the study each patient underwent an exercise test performed to maximal exertion. The patient subsequently rested for 45 min, and then repeated the effort 10 min after the administration of 0.6 mg of nitroglycerin sublingually. All patients then received in a double-blind fashion capsules of similar appearance containing either placebo or ISDN, 40 mg, which were taken orally every 8 h for 1 month. Exercise studies were repeated 6 h after the ingestion of the last capsule. These studies enabled the measurement of maximal exercise

142

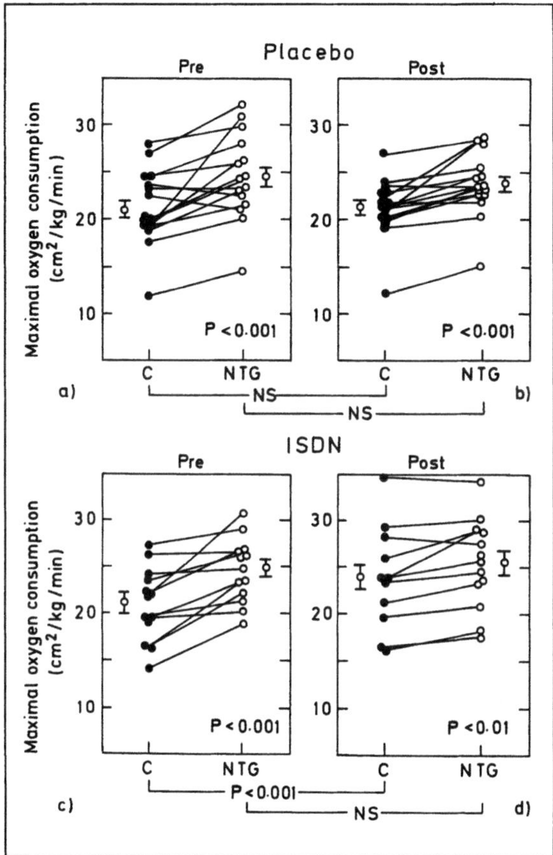

Fig. 3a–d. Group data for a derived index of oxygen consumption ($V\dot{O}_2$) before (*Pre*) and after (*Post*) 1 month of treatment with placebo or isosorbide dinitrate (*ISDN*) capsules. Prenitroglycerin control (*C*) and postnitroglycerin (*NTG*) exercise tests were performed at each period.

duration, a derived index of maximal total body oxygen consumption obtained from a regression equation by Bruce, and ST-segment depression on the electrocardiogram.

Results

All Patients manifested at least 1 mm of ST-segment depression for 60 msec on exercise electrocardiography. No significant alterations were observed in the symptoms that resulted in the termination of exercise after administration of either placebo or ISDN.

Duration of Exercise

Individual and mean data on the duration of exercise are shown in Fig. 2. During the control period in patients who received placebo (Fig. 2a), the sublingual administration of nitroglycerin prolonged the duration of exercise from 302 ± 24 to 390 ± 27 s (mean $\pm$ SEM) ($p < 0.001$). One month after placebo therapy, this group manifested an almost

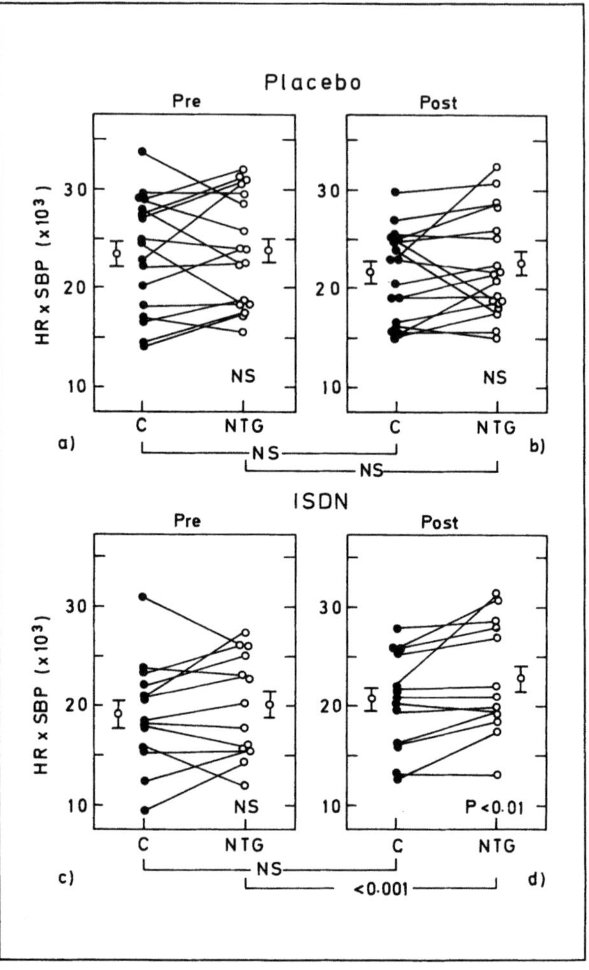

Fig. 4a–d. Group data for heart rate–systolic blood pressure product $(HR \times SBP)$ $(\times 10^3)$ before (*Pre*) and after (*Post*) 1 month of treatment with placebo or isosorbide dinitrate (*ISDN*) capsules. Prenitroglycerin control (*C*) and postnitroglycerin (*NTG*) exercise tests were performed at each period.

identical $(p > 0.05)$ increase in exercise duration from 306 ± 18 to 368 ± 20 s $(p < 0.001)$ (Fig. 2b). Thus no significant difference was observed in the increased duration of treadmill exercise after sublingually administered nitroglycerin in the patients who received placebo. Premedication exercise tests in the patients who received ISDN also demonstrated an increased duration of exercise after nitroglycerin from 302 ± 30 to 391 ± 27 s $(p < 0.001)$ (Fig. 2c). After 1 month of ISDN therapy, prenitroglycerin exercise duration in this group increased to 373 ± 36 s $(p < 0.001)$ (Fig. 2d), a value significantly higher than that of the prenitroglycerin exercise duration before ISDN therapy. Importantly, after nitroglycerin the maximal achievable duration of exertion in the group given ISDN was increased even further than before the sublingual administration of this agent, to 411 ± 34 s $(p < 0.001)$ (Fig. 2d). In addition, the maximal period of exertion after the administration of nitroglycerin was similar $(p > 0.05)$ before and after the 1-month period of ISDN therapy.

144

Maximal Oxygen Consumption Index

Data regarding the derived index of maximal oxygen consumption are given in Fig. 3. Maximal oxygen consumption improved from 21.1 ± 0.9 (prenitroglycerin) to 24.5 ± 1 (postnitroglycerin) ($p < 0.001$) (Fig. 3a) and from 21.3 ± 0.7 (prenitroglycerin) to 23.7 ± 0.8 (postnitroglycerin) cm²/kg/min ($p < 0.001$) (Fig. 3b) before and after, respectively, 1 month of placebo administration. In patients who received ISDN the increase in derived oxygen consumption after administration of nitroglycerin was similar to that of the patients who received placebo, from 21.1 ± 1.2 to 24.8 ± 1 ($p < 0.001$) (Fig. 3c) and 23.9 ± 1.4 to 25.4 ± 1.3 cm²/kg/min ($p < 0.01$) (Fig. 3d) before and after, respectively, 1 month of ISDN therapy. Thus maximal achievable derived oxygen consumption was identical ($p < 0.05$) after the administration of nitroglycerin in the periods before and after ISDN therapy. Consistent with the increase in exercise duration, derived maximal oxygen consumption during exercise before nitroglycerin was greater ($p < 0.001$) after 1 month of ISDN therapy.

Heart Rate – Blood Pressure Product

Data regarding heart rate–blood pressure product are depicted in Fig. 4. Maximal heart rate–blood pressure product, expressed to 10^3, was unchanged before and after the administration of nitroglycerin, from 23.3 ± 1.4 to 23.7 ± 1.3 ($p > 0.05$) (Fig. 4a) and from 21.6 ± 1.1 to 22.6 ± 1.2 ($p > 0.05$) (Fig. 4b) before and after, respectively, the administration of placebo capsules. Similarly, heart rate–blood pressure product at maximal exertion was not statistically different in the pre-ISDN period before and after the sublingual administration of nitroglycerin: from 19.2 ± 1.5 to 20.2 ± 1.5 ($p > 0.05$) (Fig. 4c). After isosorbide therapy, a minimal increase in the maximal level of this variable reaching statistical significance was observed after the sublingual administration of nitroglycerin: 22.8 ± 1.6 compared with the prenitroglycerin value of 20.7 ± 1.4 ($p < 0.01$) (Fig. 4d).

ST-Segment Depression

Regarding the quantity of ST-segment depression observed at maximal exertion (Fig. 5), nitroglycerin produced a significant reduction in this electrocardiographic abnormality, from 2.1 ± 0.3 to 1.3 ± 0.3 mm ($p < 0.01$) (Fig. 5a) before and after, respectively ($p < 0.001$) (Fig. 5b), 1 month of placebo. ST-segment depression at maximal exertion in the group given ISDN was similarly reduced after nitroglycerin in the premedication period, from 2.6 ± 0.2 to 1.8 ± 0.3 ($p < 0.002$) (Fig. 5c). However, the extent of ST-segment depression manifested in the prenitroglycerin exercise electrocardiogram after administration of isosorbide was substantially less than that observed in the control period before its administration. Thus, although the ST-segment depression at maximal exertion observed after nitroglycerin was identical before and after oral administration of ISDN, the maximal degree of ST-segment depression after isosorbide was similar before and after nitroglycerin: from 2.1 ± 0.4 mm prenitroglycerin to 2 ± 0.3 mm postnitroglycerin ($p > 0.05$) (Fig. 5d). Thus the ability of sublingually administered nitroglycerin

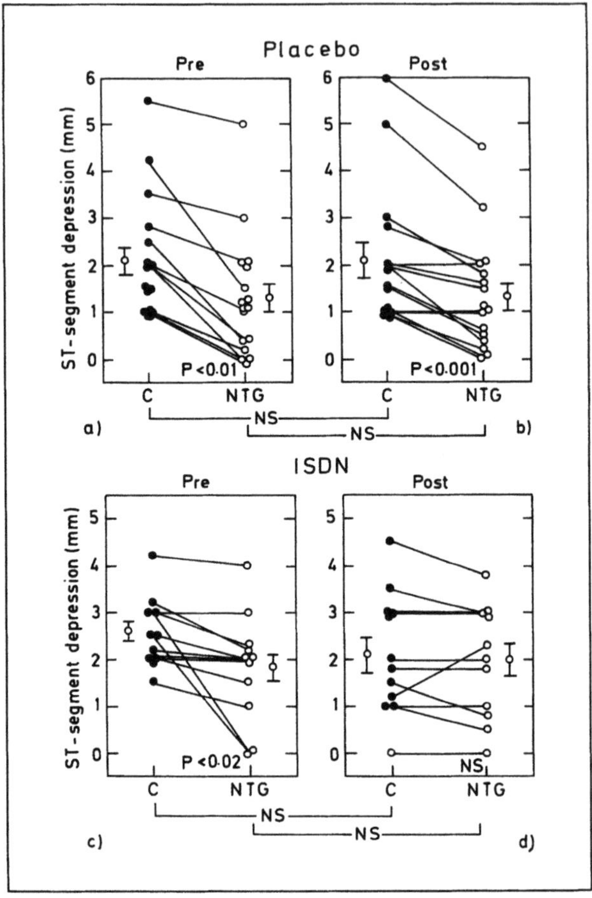

to augment exercise duration and maximal oxygen consumption without a concomitant
increase in electrocardiographic evidence of myocardial ischemia was maintained after
long-term administration of ISDN.

Percentage Alteration in Exercise Variables

Subsequently, we analyzed the percentage change from control values induced by sublingual administration of nitroglycerin in the periods before and after the administration of
placebo and ISDN. No change in the percentage increase in duration of exercise and the
derived index of oxygen consumption or the decrease in ST-segment depression induced
by nitroglycerin was observed from the pre- to postplacebo periods: from 37% to 25%,
from 17% to 12%, and from 40% to 40%, respectively (all $p > 0.05$). After administration
of ISDN, a significant augmentation of exercise duration and derived oxygen consumption and a substantial decrease in ST-segment depression were observed even before the
administration of nitroglycerin. Consequently, reductions in the percentage increase in
exercise duration induced by nitroglycerin (from 38% to 13%), derived oxygen consump-

146

tion (from 19% to 7%), and decrease in ST-segment depression (from 29% to 3%) (all $p < 0.05$) were calculated after therapy with isosorbide even though the further alterations in these variables affected by nitroglycerin resulted in values identical to those achieved in the preisosorbide period after nitroglycerin.

Discussion

Documentation of the value of orally administered sustained-release ISDN in the prophylactic therapy of angina pectoris has led to the increased application of this agent in patients with chest pain secondary to ischemic heart disease. Further, the ability to induce venous and arteriolar dilation has also led to the use of isosorbide as a ventricular unloading agent in the treatment of chronic congestive heart failure (13). Accordingly, the issue of whether ISDN induces the development of tolerance when administered orally in large doses has assumed even greater importance in recent months, especially in regard to cross-tolerance to sublingually administered nitroglycerin.
Previous studies that have evaluated the ability of long-acting organic nitrates to induce cross-tolerance to sublingual nitroglycerin have yielded conflicting results. Thus Schelling and Lasagna (14) noted a slight attenuation in the decrease in systemic blood pressure and reflex tachycardia produced by sublingual nitroglycerin after a 4-week period of pentaerythritol tetranitrate. A reduction in venodilation but not in arteriolar dilation secondary to sublingual nitroglycerin was reported by Zelis and Mason (15) using plethysmography following a 6-week period of oral administration of ISDN. Recently, Thadani and co-workers (16) conducted a complex investigation complete with plasma isosorbide levels, which demonstrated both a partial circulatory tolerance to isosorbide itself and cross-tolerance to sublingual nitroglycerin which developed rapidly. These authors suggested that this tachyphylaxis type of reaction was due to a diminution of the end organ response rather than to an accelerated metabolism of the nitrates. Opposite to these findings, Goldstein and co-workers (17) failed to observe an alteration in the response of physiologic measurements or exercise tolerance to sublingual ISDN after long-term administration; and Aronow and Chesluk (18) noted an identical antianginal effect of sublingual nitroglycerin before and after prolonged use of ISDN. The two later studies, however, were compromised by the fact that the dose of oral nitrate utilized was not as large as that required for effective prophylactic therapy of angina pectoris. Most recently, Danahy and Aronow (19) conducted a long-term (mean 5.6 months) study which failed to demonstrate either tachyphylaxis or cross-tolerance to sublingual nitroglycerin by high-dose oral ISDN.
The results of our study indicate that cross-tolerance to the antianginal effect of sublingually administered nitroglycerin is not induced by the long-term oral administration of ISDN in large doses. Maximal duration of exercise, derived index of oxygen consumption, heart rate–blood pressure product, and ST-segment depression after nitroglycerin was identical before and after long-term administration of the long-acting nitrate preparation (Figs. 2–5). Further, no major tolerance to ISDN itself was evident, since exertional capacity, oxygen consumption, and ST-segment depression were improved in the control period after 1 month of isosorbide therapy, but not after placebo. However, our study was not specifically designed to evaluate tolerance to isosorbide itself, and it is possible that minor degrees of tolerance could have been overlooked.

Isosorbide dinitrate was administered in large doses for 1 month in our study. That this period is sufficiently long to induce cross-tolerance to nitroglycerin is indicated by the finding that circulatory responsiveness to nitroglycerin was reduced in a similar period of time in two previous studies (14–15). In addition, headaches precipitated by nitrates have characteristically been observed to disappear within a few weeks (20, 21). Finally, evidence of cross-tolerance to the vasodilator effects of nitroglycerin has been recorded after only 3 days of nitrate administration in rats (22).

Data gathered previously indicating that long-term administration of long-acting organic nitrates induces cross-tolerance to nitroglycerin dealt primarily with isolated measures of cardiocirculatory function, such as systemic blood pressure and forearm venous tone (14, 15). Accordingly, few inferences regarding the influence of long-term nitrate administration upon the clinical antianginal effect of nitroglycerin could be drawn from these reports. In our investigation, exercise stress testing provided an objective method for evaluating the influence of long-term ISDN therapy on the clinical antianginal effects of nitroglycerin. Earlier studies have shown that maximal exercise capacity during treadmill-walking is readily reproducible in patients with coronary artery disease after an initial educational experience (23). The identical values recorded for both exercise duration and derived index of maximal oxygen consumption before and after placebo therapy (Figs. 2 and 3) well demonstrated that peak exertion is indeed constant. The finding that nitroglycerin induced the same duration of exercise and derived maximal oxygen consumption with equivalent ST-segment depression after and before long-acting ISDN therapy thereby provides substantial objective evidence that the latter does not induce cross-tolerance to the clinical antianginal effects of nitroglycerin.

We also analyzed our data with regard to percentage improvement in those measurements manifesting a response to sublingually administered nitroglycerin.

No differences were noted in any of the exercise functions assessed after as compared with before placebo. Conversely, reductions in the percentage increase in exercise duration and the derived index of oxygen consumption and decrease in ST-segment depression induced by nitroglycerin were observed after administration of ISDN. This diminution in the percentage change in response to nitroglycerin was referable entirely to alterations in these values produced by the sustained action of ISDN in the control period. Thus significant increases in exercise duration and derived oxygen consumption and a substantial decrease in ST-segment depression occurred prior to the administration of nitroglycerin after 1 month of isosorbide therapy. Nevertheless, nitroglycerin was still able to augment further these beneficial effects to levels identical with those produced before isosorbide administration (Fig. 5). Patients therefore continued to achieve the same maximal duration of exercise and derived oxygen consumption in response to nitroglycerin without additional ST-segment depression after ISDN therapy as before it. Our interpretation of these data was that a maximal antianginal effect could be produced by nitroglycerin, and that this maximum was achieved both prior to and following ISDN.

It has been demonstrated that, although heart rate–blood pressure product does not account for all the determinants of myocardial oxygen demand, it represents a relatively accurate index of this measure (24). Accordingly, interventions that enable greater duration of exercise and maximal oxygen demand by virtue of increasing myocardial oxygen supply (such as coronary artery bypass surgery) are associated with increases in heart rate–blood pressure product. The observation that the rate–pressure product was unchanged at maximal exertion after nitroglycerin in our study supports the concept that the in-

148

crease in exercise capacity produced by this agent is referable to a decrease in myocardial oxygen demand. Although the maximal rate–pressure product increased slightly after nitroglycerin during exercise testing after ISDN therapy, the change was considered too small to be of substantial physiological significance.

In conclusion, our data indicate that cross-tolerance to the antianginal effect of sublingually administered nitroglycerin is not induced by long-term oral administration of ISDN. Although previous studies have reported evidence suggesting the development of cross-tolerance to nitroglycerin induced by long-acting nitrates, such small changes in circulatory function apparently do not impair the clinical antianginal effect of this agent.

References

1. Goldberg AN, Moran JF, Butterfield TK et al: Therapy of angina pectoris with propranolol and long-acting nitrates. Circulation 40: 847–853 (1969).
2. Battock DJ, Alvarez H, Chidsey CA: Effects of propranolol and isosorbide dinitrate on exercise performance and adrenergic activity in patients with angina pectoris. Circulation 39: 157–169 (1969).
3. Sweatman T, Strauss G, Selzer A et al: The long-acting hemodynamic effects of isosorbide dinitrate. Am J Cardiol 29: 475–480 (1972).
4. Battock DJ, Levitt PW, Steele PP: Effects of isosorbide dinitrate and nitroglycerin on central circulatory dynamics in coronary artery disease. Am Heart J 92: 455–458 (1976).
5. Brunner D, Meshulam N, Zerieker F: Effectiveness of sustained-action isosorbide dinitrate on exercise-induced myocardial ischemia. Chest 66: 282–287 (1974).
6. Danahy DT, Burwell DT, Aronow WS et al: Sustained hemodynamic and antianginal effect of high dose oral isosorbide dinitrate. Circulation 55: 381–387 (1977).
7. Lee G, Mason DT, Amsterdam EA et al: Improved exercise tolerance for 6 hours following isosorbide dinitrate capsules in patients with ischemic heart disease (abstr). Am J Cardiol 37: 150 (1976).
8. Kasparian H, Weiner L, Duca PR et al: Comparative hemodynamic effects of placebo and oral isosorbide dinitrate in patients with significant coronary artery disease. Am Heart J 90: 68–74 (1975).
9. Glancy DL, Richter MA, Ellis EV: Effects of swallowed isosorbide dinitrate on blood pressure, heart rate and exercise tolerance in patients with coronary artery disease (abstr). Circulation 51, 52: Suppl II: II–189 (1975).
10. Fremont RE: Controlled observations on clinical efficacy of isosorbide dinitrate. Geriatrics 16: 520–529 (1961).
11. Willis WH Jr, Russell RO Jr, Mantle JA et al: Hemodynamic effects of isosorbide dinitrate vs nitroglycerin in patients with unstable angina. Chest 69: 15–22 (1976).
12. Winsor, T, Kaye H, Mills B: Hemodynamic response of long-acting nitrates: evidence of gastrointestinal absorption. Chest 62: 407–413 (1972).
13. Franciosa JA, Mikulic E, Cohn JN et al: Hemodynamic effects of orally administered isosorbide dinitrate in patients with congestive heart failure. Circulation 50: 1020–1024 (1974).
14. Schelling JL, Lasagna L: A study of cross-tolerance to circulatory effects of organic nitrates. Clin Pharmacol Ther 8: 256–260 (1967).
15. Zelis R, Mason DT: Isosorbide dinitrate. Effect on the vasodilator response to nitroglycerin. JAMA 234: 166–170 (1975).
16. Thadani U, Manyari D, Parker JO, Fung HL: Tolerance to the circulatory effects of oral isosorbide dinitrate. Rate of development and cross-tolerance to glyceryl trinitrate. Circulation 61: 526–535 (1980).
17. Goldstein RE, Rosing DR, Redwood DR et al: Clinical and circulatory effects of isosorbide dinitrate. Comparison with nitroglycerin. Circulation 43: 629–640 (1971).
18. Aronow WS, Chesluk HM: Evaluation of nitroglycerin in angina in patients on isosorbide dinitrate. Circulation 42: 61–63 (1970).

19. Danahy DT, Aronow WS: Hemodynamics and antianginal effects of high dose oral isosorbide dinitrate after chronic use. Circulation 56: 205–212 (1977).
20. Stewart DD: Tolerance to nitroglycerine. JAMA 44: 1678–1679 (1905).
21. Schwartz AM: The cause, relief, and prevention of headaches arising from contact with dynamite. N Engl J Med 235: 541–544 (1946).
22. Needleman P, Johnson EM Jr: Mechanism of tolerance development to organic nitrates. J Pharmacol Exp Ther 184: 709–715 (1973).
23. Dagenais GR, Pitt B, Ross RS: Exercise tolerance in patients with angina pectoris. Am J Cardiol 28: 10–16 (1971).
24. Robinson BF: Relation of heart rate and systolic blood pressure to the onset of pain in angina pectoris. Circulation 35: 1073–1083 (1967).

Authors' address:
Anthony N. DeMaria, M.D.
Division of Cardiovascular Medicine
University of Kentucky College of Medicine
Lexington, Kentucky 40536–0084

Discussion

FRANCIOSA:

Dr. DeMaria, your study addressed the question of a cross-tolerance between isosorbide dinitrate and nitroglycerin, I wonder if you are aware of any studies using a similar type of protocol looking at the question of tolerance of isosorbide dinitrate istself, for example using sublingual isosorbide dinitrate instead of nitroglycerin.

DeMARIA:

There are several studies that were done in the early Seventies with doses of isosorbide dinitrate of 40 mg per day which are probably no more relevant. I would like to ask Dr. Schneider, based upon his experience, if now routinely such high daily doses are used in patients with coronary heart disease.

SCHNEIDER:

Routinely our dose-levels are in the range of 120 to 160 mg per day, but if necessary we increase the daily dosage to 480 mg.

FRANCIOSA:

What ist the definition of the dose needed? Dr. Schneider's data show that even at 480 mg per day only a 50% reduction of angina could be obtained, and some of the patients were still having 6 anginal episodes per week.

SCHNEIDER:

The data showed the mean values. 5 patients were free of angina with the highest dose, but others were not markedly improved.

KALTENBACH:

Did you use a sustained-release ISDN formulation in your study?

DEMARIA:

Yes.

The Effect of Long-Acting Nitrates on Ambulatory ECG Changes in Patients with Angina Pectoris Treated for 1 Week

K. M. Fox, J. E. Deanfield, C. Wright, P. Ribeiro and A. Maseri

Introduction

Although both sublingual and inhaled nitrates have been shown to be effective, and were introduced over 100 years ago (1), it is only in very recent years that the oral nitrates have been shown to be effective in the treatment of angina pectoris (2, 3). Even today considerable controversy still exists as to exactly how effective these drugs are when taken as chronic therapy. Tolerance to nitrates is well known (4), and recent studies have shown attenuation of hemodynamic effects even by the fifth oral dose (5). Many of the difficulties arise because the effects of nitrates in angina has been objectively assessed using acute hemodynamic studies such as exercise testing (6). There have been no objective evaluations of the drug in the daily life of patients with angina. Although anginal frequency and glyceryl trinitrate consumption are important guides to therapy, they probably only represent the tip of the iceberg in terms of the number of episodes of transient myocardial ischemia these patients are experiencing (7).

The introduction of ambulatory monitoring has added a new dimension to the objective evaluation of patients with angina pectoris (8). Provided patients are carefully selected, the frequency of ST-segment depression can be used as an objective evaluation of the occurrence of myocardial ischemia. This study was designed to determine the effects of oral administration of ISDN on the frequency of myocardial ischemia in patients with chronic stable angina pectoris.

Patients and Methods

Patients:

Ten patients were studied. These were nine males and one female. All patients had chronic stable angina known to occur both at rest and on exertion and to have at least one episode of angina per day. All patients had a positive exercise test and all other causes of ST-segment depression were excluded. In addition, in all patients exercise-induced ST-segment depression was shown to reflect myocardial ischemia using radionuclide techniques (rubidium-82 + positron emission tomography) (9).

Methods:

The trial was double-blind. Each patient underwent five 1-week treatment periods. Three of these treatments were placebo and two were active ISDN treatments (one comprising

40 mg four times a day, and the other 160 mg once a day (Isoket)). A double dummy technique was employed and the design of the study was such that each active phase was followed by a placebo phase.

Measurements:

Ambulatory monitoring was performed both during the first 48 h of each treatment other than the first and during the last 2 days of each treatment. Ambulatory monitoring of ST segments was performed using an Oxford Medilog II analyzer together with Oxford Medilog frequency-modulated recording boxes. Each tape was analyzed visually at times 60 speed by two independent and experienced observers. In each 24-h period the number of episodes of ST-segment depression, the duration of each episode, and the time each episode occurred were noted. An episode was only considered to be present when there was at least 1 ml planar ST-segment depression occurring 0.08 s after the end of the QRS complex.

Results

The results of the study are shown in Figs. 1 and 2. Figure 1 shows the number of episodes and duration of ST-segment depression in the two placebo and two active phases recorded over the first 48 h of each treatment. It can be seen that there were no significant

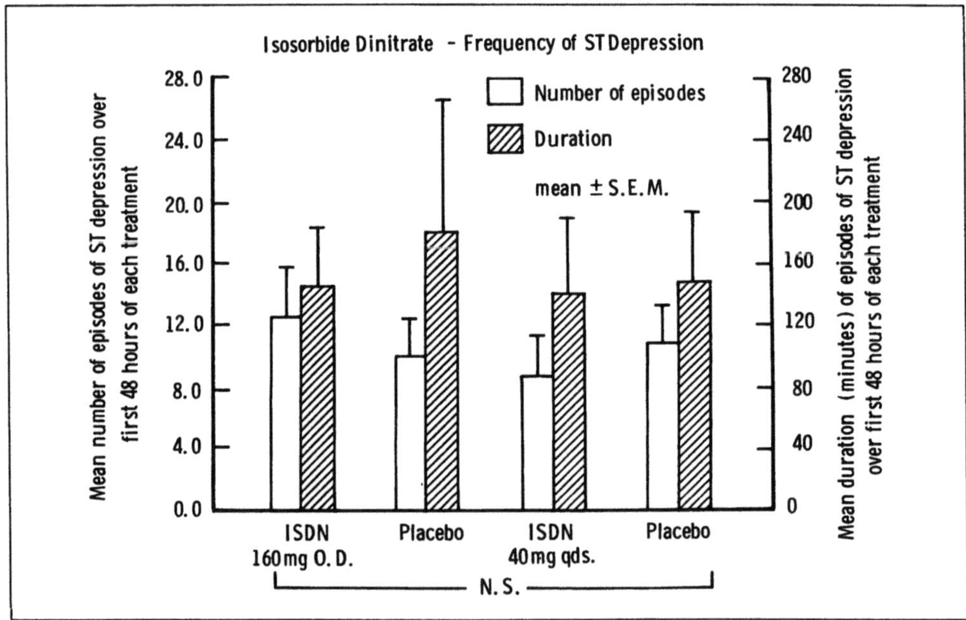

Fig. 1. The number and duration of the episodes of ST-segment depression recorded over the first 48 h of each treatment. No significant differences were found between the placebo and active phases of the treatment. *ISDN,* isosorbide dinitrate; *OD,* once daily; *qds,* four times daily.

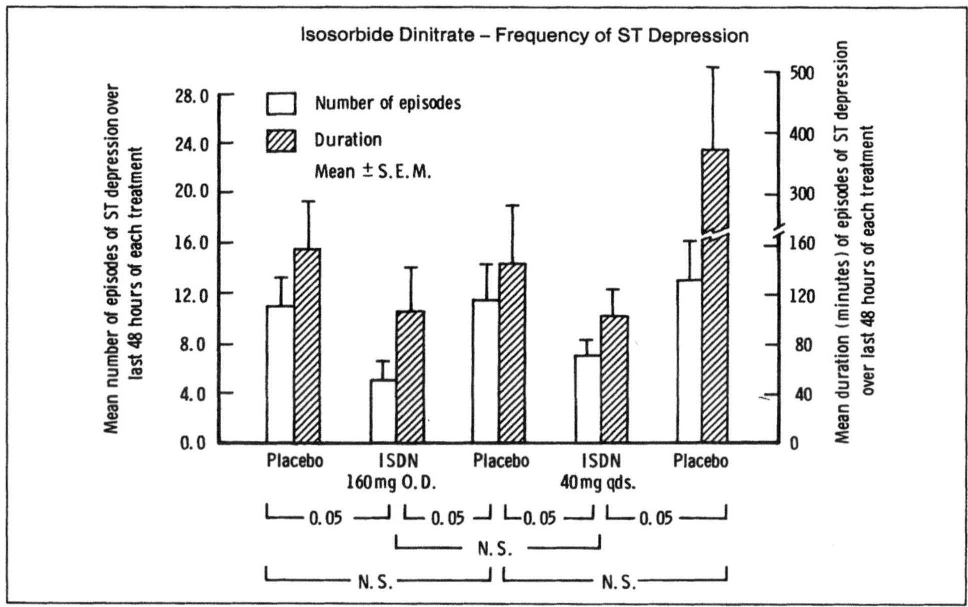

Fig. 2. The mean number and duration of episodes of ST-segment depression recorded over the last 48 h of each week's treatment. Both forms of treatment were associated with a significant reduction in the number and duration of episodes of ST-segment depression. *ISDN*, isosorbide dinitrate; *OD*, once daily; *qds*, four times daily.

differences between the two active and two placebo treatments. In contrast, at the end of 1 week of treatment, with both ISDN 40 mg four times a day and ISDN 160 mg a day there was a significant reduction in both the number of episodes of ST-segment depression and their duration. No significant differences were seen between the two active periods or the three placebo periods.

Discussion

The aims of this study were to determine: (a) whether long-acting nitrates can influence the number of episodes and the duration of ST-segment changes in patients with angina; (b) whether this effect is evident in the first 48 h of treatment and/or during the last 48 h of 1 week's treatment; (c) whether there was any rebound following the sudden cessation of treatment; and (d) whether there was any difference between the effects of ISDN given orally in sustained-release form four times a day and ISDN given orally in a single sustained-release dose each day.

The study showed that by the end of 1 week's treatment both forms of ISDN caused significant reduction in a number of episodes of ST-segment depression. This was associated with a significant reduction in the duration of these episodes. No effect was seen, however, in the first 48 h of treatment. The reason why an effect was seen in the last and not the first 48 h is not immediately clear, but possibly reflects the fact that the cumulative effect of chronic dosing is necessary to prevent myocardial ischemia with oral nitrates.

An important feature in the design of this study was the use of five placebo periods of 48 h over the 5 weeks of study. If ambulatory monitoring is to be used to evaluate drug treatment it is essential to ensure the stability of the disease. During the five placebo periods the number of episodes of ST-segment depression and their duration were relatively stable; we can thus be confident that the changes seen were due to the drugs and not due to spontaneous variation in the disease itself.

Great care was taken in selecting the patients. Frequent but stable angina was a prerequisite for entry to the study. Furthermore, all patients had a positive exercise test showing ST-segment changes to reflect myocardial ischemia. Only so can it be assumed that the ST-segment changes seen on ambulatory monitoring truly reflect myocardial ischemia.

No rebound was seen when the oral nitrates were discontinued. There were no significant differences between the two preparations of oral nitrates.

In summary, long-acting nitrates were shown significantly to reduce the number and duration of episodes of ST-segment depression recorded in ambulatory patients at the end of 1 week's treatment, though the effect was not evident in the first 48 h of treatment.

Summary

Ten patients with chronic stable but frequent angina pectoris were studied. Each patient underwent five 1-week treatment periods consisting of three placebo and two active treatments. The two active treatments were isosorbide dinitrate (ISDN) 40 mg four times a day and ISDN 160 mg a day, both in sustained-release preparations. Randomization was such that each active treatment was followed by a placebo phase. The study was double-blind and ambulatory monitoring of ST segments was performed for 48 h at the beginning and end of each treatment. Both preparations of ISDN were found similarly to reduce the number and duration of episodes of ST-segment depression at the end of 1 week's treatment. This effect was not evident in the first 48 h. No rebound was seen to occur when the drugs were stopped.

References

1. Murrel W: Nitroglycerin as a remedy for angina pectoris. Lancet 1: 80 (1979).
2. Danahy DT, Burwell DT, Aronow WS, Prakash R: Sustained hemodynamic and antianginal effect of high dose oral isosorbide dinitrate. Circulation 55: 381–387 (1977).
3. Markis J, Gorlin R, Mills RM, Williams RA, Schweitzel P, Ransil BJ: Sustained effect of orally administered isosorbide dinitrate on exercise performance of patients with angina pectoris. Am J Cardiol 43: 265–267 (1979).
4. Needleman P, Johnson EM Jr: Mechanism of tolerance development to organic nitrates. J Pharmacol and experiment therapeut 184: 709–715 (1973).
5. Thadani U, Manyari D, Parker JO, Fung H: Tolerance to the circulatory effects of oral isosorbide dinitrate. Rate of development and cross tolerance to glyceryl trinitrate. Circulation 61: 526–535 (1980).
6. Lee G, Mason DT, DeMaria AN: Effects of long term oral administration of isosorbide dinitrate on the antianginal response to nitroglycerin. Absence of nitrate cross tolerance and self tolerance shown by exercise testing. Am J Cardiol 41: 82–87 (1978).
7. Schang SJ, Pepine CJ: Transient asymptomatic ST segment depression during daily activity. Am J of Cardiol 39: 396–402 (1977).

8. Selwyn AP, Fox K, Eves M, Oakley D, Dargie H, Shillingford JP: Myocardial ischemia in patients with frequent angina pectoris. Brit Med J 2: 1594–1596 (1978).
9. Selwyn AP, Allan RM, Fox KM, Horlock P, O'Brian H, Maseri A: Prolonged myocardial ischemia in angina. Circulation 64: IV-82 1981 (abstract).

Authors' address:
Dr. K. M. Fox
Cardiovascular Unit
Hammersmith Hospital
Du Cane Road
London W12 OHS

Discussion

GLEICHMANN:

You said the main effects were seen in patients with slow heart rates. Did you differentiate between the duration, the influence on the anginal attacks during daytime and during the night? Maybe among your group there were more cases with Prinzmetal angina?

FOX:

Quite a number of our patients had episodes of ST-segment depression at night. I don't think they fulfil the criteria of typical Prinzmetal angina. Our belief is that the majority of patients who have frequent myocardial ischaemia do in fact show episodes at night, perhaps in the early morning hours. We haven't specifically distinguished between episodes during day and night. We have just looked at the heart rate effect. All I can comment on, is that isosorbide dinitrate is active at the end of one week and appeared to have maximum effects in patients with slow heart rate.

ABRAMS:

I see correlations between the dosage of ISDN and the effects and would like to ask you for a comment on the difference in the dosage in your study compared to Dr. Schneider's study, where some of the statistically significant effects, particularly on the number of anginal attacks, were only seen at very high doses up to 480 mg per day.

FOX:

We used 4 × 40 mg of ISDN.

ABRAMS:

Dr. Fox used what some of us would consider low-dose isosorbide dinitrate and Dr. Schneider's work suggested that the maximum effect could be obtained only with much higher dosages. Was there a difference in the ratio of symptomatic versus asymptomatic episodes of ST-segment depression? This would indicate that ISDN could prevent anginal pain during episodes with ST-segment depression.

FOX:

Most physicians in the U.K. certainly would have considered that 160 mg a day of the slow-release preparation was a reasonable dose, but perhaps in view of certain results one should go to higher doses.
To answer the second question, we haven't analyzed our data in that way.

BUSSMANN:

I should like to point out the large variations of the ST-segment changes in the placebo group. In one placebo period many episodes of ST-segment depression have been found and in the other placebo period the incidence was very low.

FOX:

The results in the placebo groups in fact were remarkably constant. The difference was due to a very long episode of angina in one patient of the third placebo group. But there was actually no significant difference in any of the placebo groups at either the beginning or the end. All placebo groups were very similar.
I should like to further specify that the second exercise test was done 55 minutes after the first one, there was a 45 minutes rest period, then nitrates were administered. We then waited 10 minutes to get a maximal effect. A very interesting question is how long ischaemia persists. We are dealing with so many different manifestations of ischaemia. In wall motion studies with nuclear techniques the measurements have to be performed within the first 5 or 10 minutes after the termination of exercise. After this period the wall motion will have returned to normal. In our study we measured 20 minutes after administration, but found metabolic rather than wall motion changes.

DEMARIA:

The technique used has therefore to be considered. There are two questions: how many patients were investigated and were the patients physically more active during ISDN treatment than prior to treatment?

FOX:

The reason we only studied 10 patients was that the design was quite rigorous. Each patient had 2 days of ambulatory monitoring at the beginning and 2 days at the end of each 7-day period. Only during the weekend there was no monitoring. The patients kept a diary, but it is difficult to be sure whether they did more activities. Also, some of the patients find it very difficult to distinguish between various kinds of pain, they find it difficult to decide which chest pain is angina and which is not. That is why we wanted to concentrate on the ambulatory monitoring. It is possible that the patients could have done more work in the first 48 hours. On the other hand, the efficacy of the drug could be less during the first hours than later on. It is not the blood level that is important, but the tissue concentration of the nitrate. It may take time until tissue concentrations are high enough to prevent ischemic episodes.

STAUCH:

Referring to your statement about rubidium uptake after 20 minutes, I want to ask you whether you could characterize the patients in some closer way, maybe from angiographic studies. We have found in studies with radionuclide ventriculography that occasionally changes in wall motion did not return to normal after 20 minutes, but often react very promptly to nitrates. These seem to be the patients who have very diffuse coronary heart disease.

FOX:

The patients we are studying are patients with severe three-vessel disease. Although we do see patients who have frequent episodes of ST-segment depression and normal coronary arteries, the majority of patients do have severe three-vessel-disease. Not only the type of ischaemia but also the severity of ischaemia seem to be in some way related to the time it takes for recovery. For instance, we find that the rubidium defects returned to normal much quicker after a cold pressure test than after a maximal exercise test.

Chronic Treatment of Ischemic Heart Disease with Isosorbide Dinitrate Retard Tablets: Evidence of Preserved Hemodynamic Response to a Sublingual Dose of 5 mg

A. Distante, E. Moscarelli, M. A. Morales, M. Lombardi, C. Palombo, F. Sabino, and A. L'Abbate

Introduction

Recent clinical experiences have suggested that high doses of nitrates administered by continuous infusion are very effective both in relieving pain and in preventing myocardial ischemic attacks in patients with frequent anginal episodes at rest (1–2). However, intravenous therapy cannot be proposed for long-term treatment and different routes of administration (sublingual, oral, or percutaneous) are usually employed for chronic use in outpatients.

On the other hand, the chronic use of nitrates has been reported to lead to circulatory tolerance, as documented by an attenuation of the hemodynamic responsiveness over time to acute additional doses of the same drug (3–7). Nevertheless, this conclusion has been contradicted by the results of others (8–10). The purpose of this study was to evaluate the possible development of circulatory tolerance to nitrates in patients under chronic oral

Table 1. Clinical, electrocardiographic, and angiographic characteristics of patient population (N = 48)

Angina	On effort	8
	At rest	15
	At rest + on effort	25
Stress test ECG	Not recorded	14
	Normal	16
	Abnormal	18
ECG during pain	Not recorded	20
	Normal	7
	Abnormal	21
Ventriculography	Not recorded	11
	Normal	14
	Abnormal	23
Coronary Angiography	Not recorded	11
	Normal	3
	Abnormality in one vessels	4
	Abnormality in two vessels	17
	Abnormality in three vessels	13

treatment with isosorbide dinitrate (ISDN), as judged by the hemodynamic response to an additional test dose of the same drug given sublingually.

Materials and Methods
Selection of Patients

We selected 48 patients (40 males and 8 females aged from 36 to 78 [mean 54.8] years) who had been admitted to hospital because of frequent anginal attacks. Of these, 25 complained of anginal pain both at rest and on effort, 15 patients only had angina at rest, and 8 patients had angina only on effort. Clinical, electrocardiographic, and angiographic characteristics of the patients are summarized in Table 1.
No patient had clinical or biochemical signs of renal or hepatic dysfunction.
Thirty-eight patients were under associated treatment with verapamil to potentiate the antianginal effects of nitrates; 11 patients were on treatment with digitalis to prevent cardiac failure and one was also on beta-blocking therapy; 16 patients were periodically on diuretics to prevent heart failure or mild hypertension.
After clinical evaluation and selected diagnostic procedures performed at hospital admission, all these patients were treated in hospital and after discharge with ISDN oral tablets at a dose ranging from 60 to 240 mg daily (mean 100 mg) in three doses.

Protocol of the Study

Patients studied were under chronic continuous treatment with ISDN (for 1–60 months, average 21 months). All patients were on therapy the day of the trial, the last dose having been administered 2–6 h before the acute study. Patientes were kept in a supine position while electrocardiographic and cuff blood pressure were obtained every minute.
When heart rate and blood pressure values showed no significant fluctuation and always following 15 min rest, 5 mg ISDN was administered sublingually. Heart rate and systolic and diastolic blood pressure were measured every minute for at least 10 min after ISDN administration. No patient was studied during an anginal attack or during symptoms of heart failure. The absolute values of maximal changes in these three parameters and their values as percentages of control were considered. All the patients were told of the reasons for the trial and gave their informed consent to the study.

Statistical Analysis

For statistical analysis patients were either considered as a whole population or divided into five groups according to the duration of the chronic treatment. Classic statistical methods (correlation, variance, Student's t-test) were used to evaluate the relation between duration of treatment and hemodynamic response to the test dose in the entire population as well as to compare the hemodynamic response in each group of patients.

Table 2. Mean values and their standard errors for heart rate (HR), systolic blood pressure (SBP), and diastolic blood pressure (DBP)

Group	No. of patients	Months (mean + SEM)	HR (mean + SEM)		SBP (mean + SEM)		DBP (mean + SEM)	
			Basal	Max response	Basal	Max response	Basal	Max response
A	5	4 ± 0.9	73.2 ± 4.6	75.4 ± 5.6 4.6 ± 1.1 % (2.8 ± 2.9)	140 ± 13	124 ± 11.6 −16 ± 3.3 %(−10.2 ± 2.2)	85.6 ± 4.1	81.8 ± 5 −3.8 ± 2.5 %(−4.5 ± 2.9)
B	11	10.6 ± 0.5	70.6 ± 3	79.7 ± 3.8 9.9 ± 1.3 %(12.7 ± 1.4)	144 ± 7.2	124.7 ± 4.5 −19.3 ± 6.7 %(−12.6 ± 3.3)	88.4 ± 4.7	81.1 ± 2.7 −7.4 ± 4.5 %(−6.7 ± 3.9)
C	9	19.5 ± 0.7	69.6 ± 4.8	78.6 ± 4.7 9 ± 1.5 %(13.7 ± 2.8)	142 ± 6.6	131.1 ± 6.9 −11.6 ± 1.3 % (−7.8 ± 1)	90.7 ± 4.1	87.4 ± 4.5 −8.1 ± 0.9 %(−1.2 ± 3.3)
D	15	24.4 ± 0.3	68.8 ± 2.3	74.1 ± 2.3 5.3 ± 0.9 % (5.6 ± 1.6)	141 ± 3.7	130.8 ± 4 −12.1 ± 2.4 % (−8.1 ± 1.7)	86.2 ± 2.6	84 ± 2.9 −2.2 ± 1.4 %(−3.9 ± 2.3)
E	8	40.5 ± 3.1	72.6 ± 3.8	80.1 ± 5.2 7.5 ± 3 %(10.3 ± 4.2)	161 ± 12.5	143.1 ± 11.1 −17.7 ± 3.9 %(−10.6 ± 2.2)	98.5 ± 6	89.2 ± 5.2 −9.2 ± 1.6 %(−9.1 ± 1.3)
A–E	48	20.9 ± 1.7	70.4 ± 0.1	77.4 ± 1.7 6.9 ± 0.8 % (9.9 ± 1.1)	145.4 ± 3.4	130.8 ± 3 −14.3 ± 1.9 % (−9.6 ± 1.1)	89.5 ± 0.1	84.8 ± 1.7 −4.5 ± 1.3 %(−5.2 ± 1.2)

Table 3. Correlations between groups in terms of heart rate (HR), systolic blood pressure (SBP), and diastolic blood pressure (DBP). DOF = degree of freedom.

Cor-relations	DOF	HR		SBP		DBP	
		t	p	t	p	t	p
A vs B	14	−3.45	< 0.01	0.26	NS	0,36	NS
A vs C	12	−2.44	< 0.05	−1.1	NS	−0,23	NS
A vs D	18	−1	NS	−0.98	NS	−0.57	NS
A vs E	11	−1.27	NS	−0.02	NS	1.61	NS
B vs C	18	−0.33	NS	−1.03	NS	−0.64	NS
B vs D	24	2.45	< 0.05	−1.46	NS	−1.08	NS
B vs E	17	−0.6	NS	−0.34	NS	0.5	NS
C vs D	22	2.18	< 0.05	−0.33	NS	0.7	NS
C vs E	15	0.67	NS	1.06	NS	2.08	NS
D vs E	21	−0.99	NS	1	NS	2.5	< 0.02

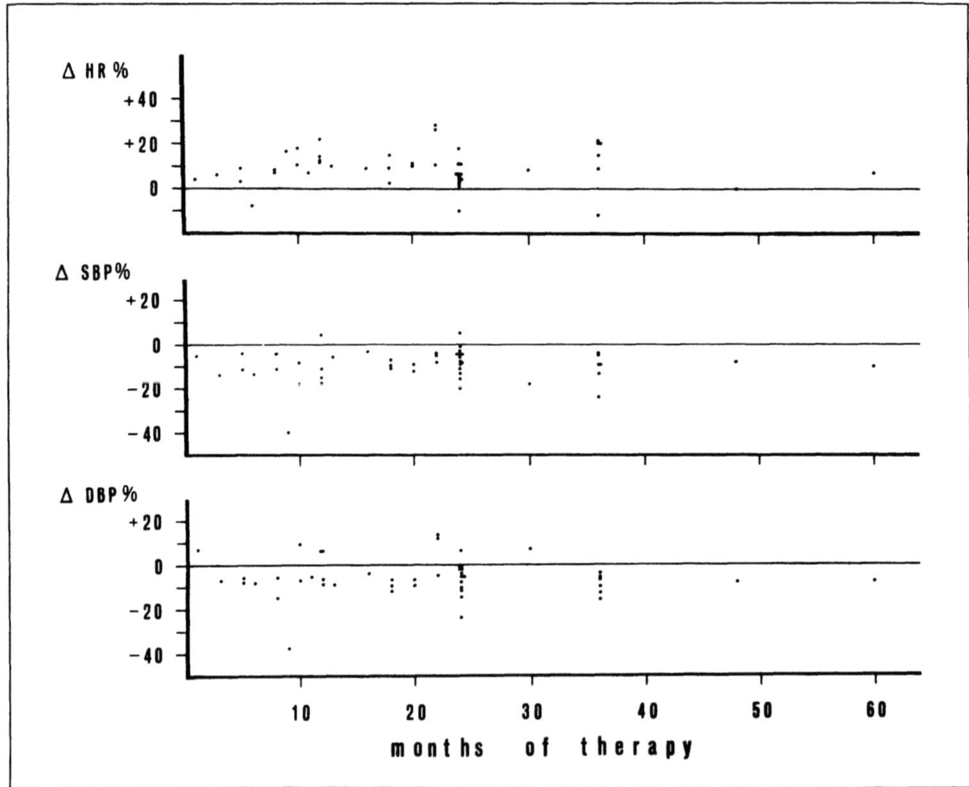

Fig. 1. Individual hemodynamic response to the test dose expressed as percentage change from basal values. *HR*, heart rate; *SBP*, systolic blood pressure; *DBP*, diastolic blood pressure.

Table 4. Correlations between duration of treatment and changes in heart rate (HR), systolic blood pressure (SBP), and diastolic blood pressure (DBP) for the groups. DOF = degree of freedom.

Group		DOF	t	r	p
A	Time vs HR	3	−0.793	−0.416	NS
B	Time vs HR	9	0.813	0.262	NS
C	Time vs HR	7	2.311	0.658	NS
D	Time vs HR	13	0.448	0.123	NS
E	Time vs HR	6	−0.694	−0.273	NS
A	Time vs SBP	3	−0.676	−0.363	NS
B	Time vs SBP	9	0.855	0.274	NS
C	Time vs SBP	7	0.364	0.136	NS
D	Time vs SBP	13	−1.695	−0.425	NS
E	Time vs SBP	6	0.238	0.097	NS
A	Time vs DBP	3	−2.949	−0.862	NS
B	Time vs DBP	9	1.27	0.39	NS
C	Time vs DBP	7	1.205	0.414	NS
D	Time vs DBP	13	1.303	0.34	NS
E	Time vs DBP	6	0.358	0.145	NS

Results

Patients were divided into five groups according to the duration of treatment (1–7, 8–14, 15–22, 23–30, or 35–60 months, the numbers of patients being 5, 11, 9, 15, and 8 respectively).

Table 2 summarizes the mean values and their standard errors for heart rate and systolic and diastolic blood pressure, both in absolute terms and as percentage changes from basal values, for the five groups and for the entire population.

When the data are considered as a block a significant hemodynamic response to sublingual administration of 5 mg ISDN was present, as assessed by the increase in heart rate and decrease in systolic and diastolic blood pressure relative to control values ($p < 0.01$ for each parameter).

When each group was compared with all other groups and the significance of difference analyzed by simultaneous Student's t-test (correction of error rate according to Bonferroni's rule [13–15]), no statistically significant differences in hemodynamic response were present between groups (Table 3). The only exception is heart rate response in group A relative to group B, the tachycardic response at 10.6 months (group B) being significantly higher ($p < 0.1$) than the one at 4 months (group A), which is the opposite of what is expected in the case of tolerance development.

Individual hemodynamic response to the test dose expressed as percentage change relative to basal values is reported for the whole population in Fig. 1. There was no significant attenuation in tachycardic and hypotensive response either in patients treated for a few months or in those treated for several months, as assessed by the absence of a correlation between duration of treatment and hemodynamic changes (r values are: − 0.003, + 0.072, and − 0.041 respectively for heart rate and systolic and diastolic blood pressure).

In Table 4 the correlations between length of treatment and changes relative to each hemodynamic parameter are given for the five groups.

Discussion

The role of nitrates in the therapy of anginal pain has been rather predominant since the discovery of Murrel and Brunton (11–12). Over time, although they are effective in clinical cardiology, their role has been questioned partly because of the lack of an ideal mode of administration and partly because of the suggestion that circulatory tolerance may develop after chronic treatment with nitrates (3–7).

Recently, following reports that a great majority of anginal attacks at rest are caused by coronary vasospasm, the role of nitrates has been greatly stressed because of their vasodilating effect on large coronary vessels. Accordingly, it has been shown that high intravenous doses of ISDN abolish or reduce the daily number of vasospastic ischemic episodes at rest (1–2). On the basis of this experience, we are currently keeping patients with anginal attacks at rest on chronic treatment with high doses of nitrates orally or percutaneously.

In this study it is shown that in patients under long-term oral treatment with ISDN there is no attenuation of hemodynamic response to 5 mg ISDN sublingually (the dose commonly used to relieve anginal pain). In fact, a hemodynamic response has been consistently observed both in patients treated for only a few months (groups A and B) and in patients treated for several months (groups C, D, and E) as assessed by an increase in heart rate and a decrease in systolic and diastolic blood pressure.

Previous authors (3–7) have documented the development of tolerance to high dosage of long-acting nitrates, while in the same studies they admit that the antianginal effect appears to be independent of the development of circulatory tolerance (incidentally, these observations support the hypothesis of a direct effect of nitrates on large coronary arteries).

The concept behind most studies on circulatory tolerance to nitrates is that the undisputed efficacy of these drugs in the acute treatment of angina pectoris is related to the reduction of the arteriolar and venous tone, that is the reduction both in afterload and in ventricular volume. According to this concept, the efficacy of nitrates would diminish during chronic therapy if such peripheral effects were attenuated or even abolished by the development of tolerance.

This assumption does not appear to be validated by previous studies, which show that, except in a minority of patients with an extremely low coronary reserve in whom nitrates may work by reducing the myocardial oxygen requirement, these drugs are effective mainly because of their ability to decrease tonus in the large coronary arteries. Thus the antianginal effect of nitrates cannot be evaluated on the basis of, or considered equivalent to, the magnitude of the systemic circulatory changes they produce, which in this study are in any case unaffected even after several months of continuous therapy.

References

1. Distante A, Maseri A, Severi S, Biagini A, Chierchia S: Management of vasospastic angina at rest with continuous infusion of ISDN. Am J Cardiol 44: 533–539 (1979).

 2. Mikolich RJ, Nicolof NB, Robinson PH, Logue BR: Relief of refractory angina with continuous intravenous infusion of nitroglycerin. Chest 77: 3, 375–379 (1980).
 3. Schelling JL, Lasagna L: A study of cross tolerance to circulatory effects of organic nitrates. Clin Pharmacol and Therapeut 8: 2, 256–260 (1967).
 4. Needleman P: Tolerance to the vascular effects of glyceryl trinitrate. J Pharmacol and Experiment Therapeut 171: 98–102 (1970).
 5. Needleman P, Johnson EM: Mechanism of tolerance development to organic nitrates. J Pharmacol and Experiment Therapeut 184: 3, 709–715 (1973).
 6. Danahy DT, Aronow WS: Hemodynamics and antianginal effects of high dose oral ISDN after chronic use. Circulation 56: 2, 205–212 (1977).
 7. Thadani U, Manyari D, Parker JO, Fung HL: Tolerance to the circulatory effects of oral ISDN. Circulation 61: 3, 526–535 (1980).
 8. Franciosa JA, Cohn JN: Sustained hemodynamic effects without tolerance during long-term ISDN treatment of chronic left ventricular failure. Am J Cardiol 45: 648–654 (1980).
 9. Sweatman T, Strauss G, Selzer A, Cohn KE: The long-acting hemodynamic effects of ISDN. Am J Cardiol 29: 475–480 (1972).
10. Goldstein RE, Rosing DR, Redwood DR, Beiser GD, Epstein SE: Clinical and circulatory effects of ISDN. Circulation 63: 629–640 (1971).
11. Brunton TL: On the use of amyl nitrite in angina pectoris. Lancet 2: 97 (1867).
12. Murrel W: Nitroglycerin as a remedy for angina pectoris. Lancet 1: 80 (1879).
13. Salvi F, Chiandotto B (Edt): Biometria, principi e metodi. Piccin Publ (1978).
14. Miller RG jr: Simultaneous statistical inference. Mc Graw Hill Publ. N.Y. (1966).
15. Dunn OJ, Clark VA: Applied statistics: analysis of variance and regression. Wiley and Sons Publ. N.Y. (1974).

Author's address:
Dr. A. Distante
Istituto di Fisiologia Clinica, C.N.R.
via Savi, 8
56100 Pisa
Italy

Discussion

KALTENBACH:

I think the problem of nitrate tolerance is difficult in itself. We add to this by raising the problem of ISDN absorption through the skin, mainly if the dose applied to the skin is not higher than that applied by the oral route.

KOBER:

Did you measure plasma concentrations and objective parameters of the action of the ointment?

DISTANTE:

We did not measure plasma concentrations, but we do behave like pragmatic people when we treat anginal patients, and without resorting to the very interesting studies and methods to detect ischaemia, we have been following patients in the hospital and outside the hospital; in the hospital by ECG monitoring and in outpatient cases by self-monitoring. Of course, symptomatology and general condition of the patients were taken into consideration. Our experience showed us that the concept used to maximize the benefits of nitrate therapy is working. In many cases we add calcium antagonists. Patients are well controlled even on high doses nitrates alone. And as we did not have what we may be call unsuccessful treatments, we saw no need to measure plasma concentrations during our study. If we look at improvements in ST-segment changes and symptomatology we believe that these patients were on a drug which was effective for them.

FRANCIOSA:

Perhaps I can comment on the plasma concentrations after topical ISDN. In a study we completed patients were given intravenous and topical ISDN in cross-over order, and we found that on the average about 30% of the ointment was absorbed compared to the intravenous dose, so I tend to believe that although the ointment absorption can be quite variable, by and large it is quite well available.

WOODCOCK:

I think that in addition to the possible problem of absorption of an ointment, there is also a compliance factor. What were your impressions on the compliance of your patients on this long-term treatment?

DISTANTE:

In Italy we do not have ISDN ointment available at pharmacies, and we have to ask Pharma Schwarz to provide us with ointment, because we are just not able to switch patients on oral ISDN once they have been on ointment. This fact in itself implies good patient compliance and long-term efficacy of the ISDN ointment as well.

Subject Index

Basic Research in
Cardiology

Archiv für Kreislaufforschung
Official Journal of the German Association of Cardiovascular Research

Initiated by Bruno Kisch — Founded by Eberhard Koch
Continued by Franz Loogen and Konrad Spang
Editors: R. Jacob, Tübingen; W. Schaper, Bad Nauheim

Subscription Information

ISSN 0300-8428
Published bimonthly
Subscription rate: DM 410,— plus mailing charge.
Single issues DM 75,—

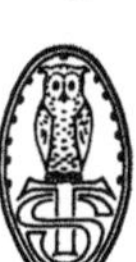

Ask for a sample copy!
Please place your order with your bookseller or send to

Dr. D. Steinkopff Verlag, P. O. Box 11 10 08, D-6100 Darmstadt